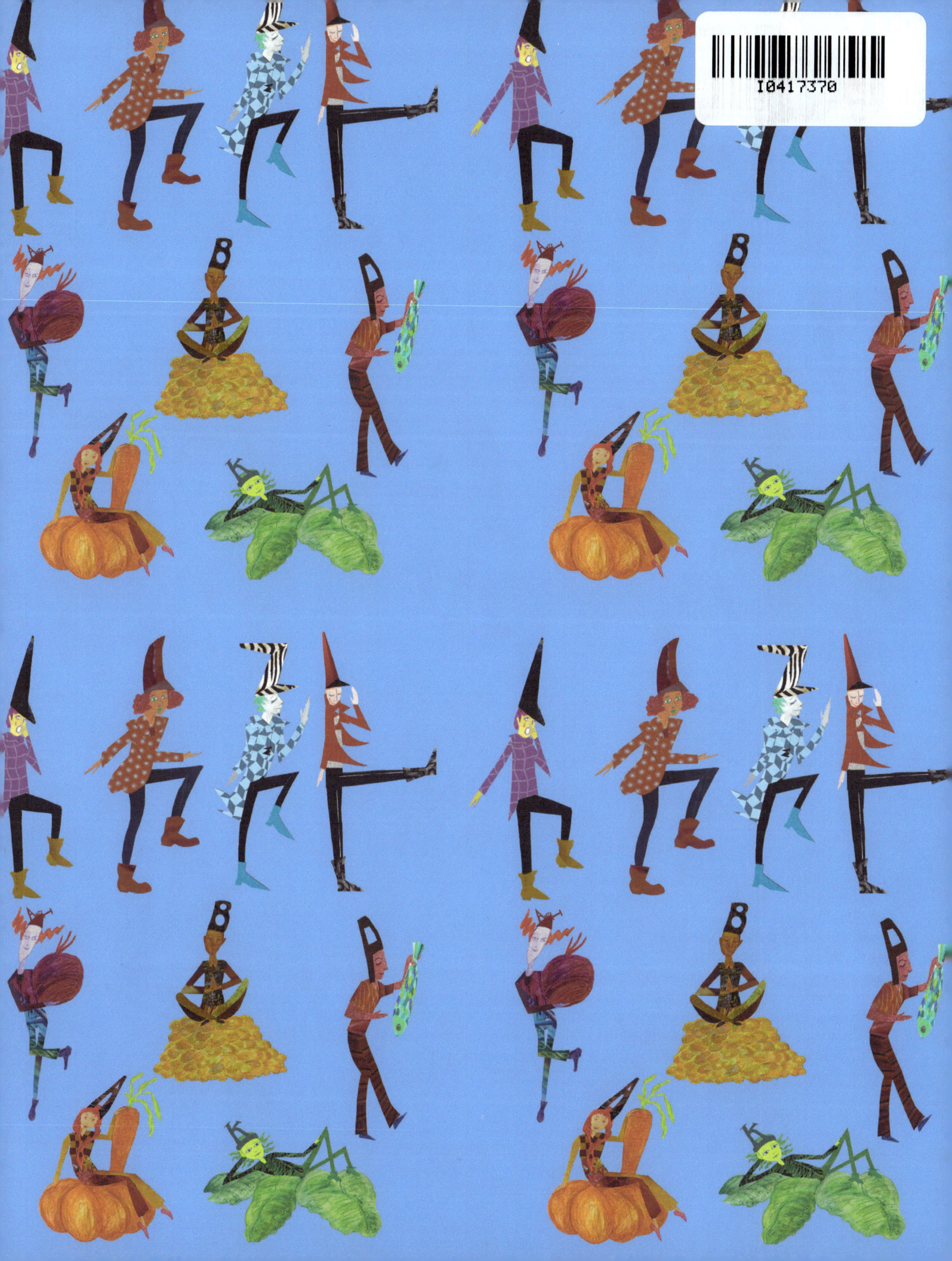

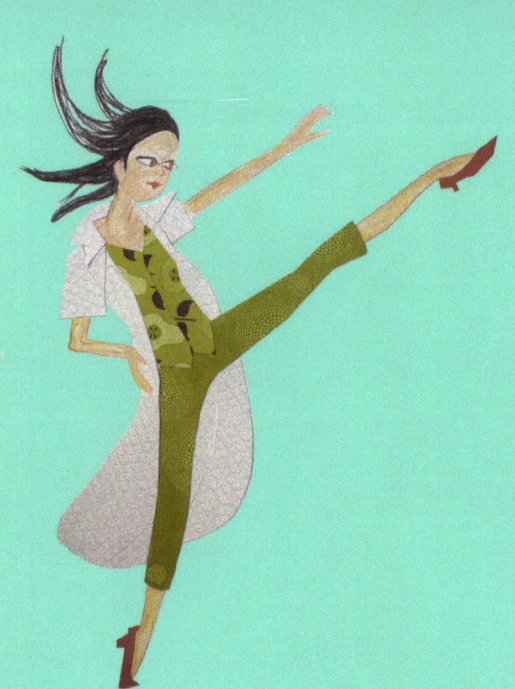

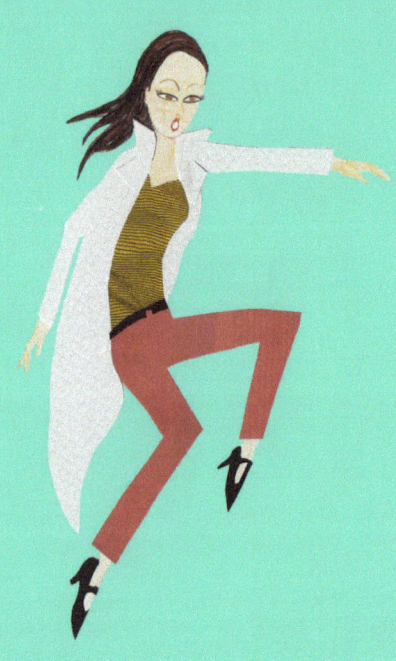

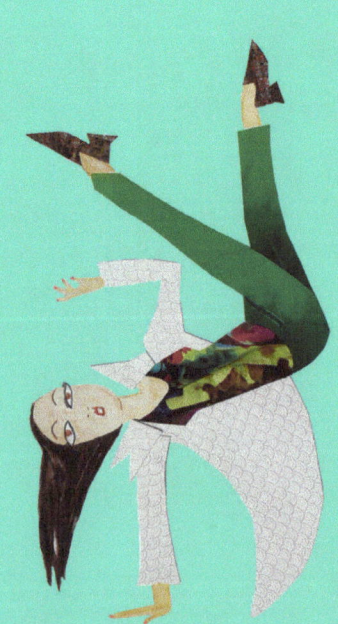

Original Edition: ©2016 Silvana Soriano & Debora Duro
Title of the Collection : Adventures of Doctor Deb
Title :The Magical Glasses
Silvana Soriano & Debora Duro
Illustration Silvana Soriano
Translation to English Clarisse Bandeira de Mello

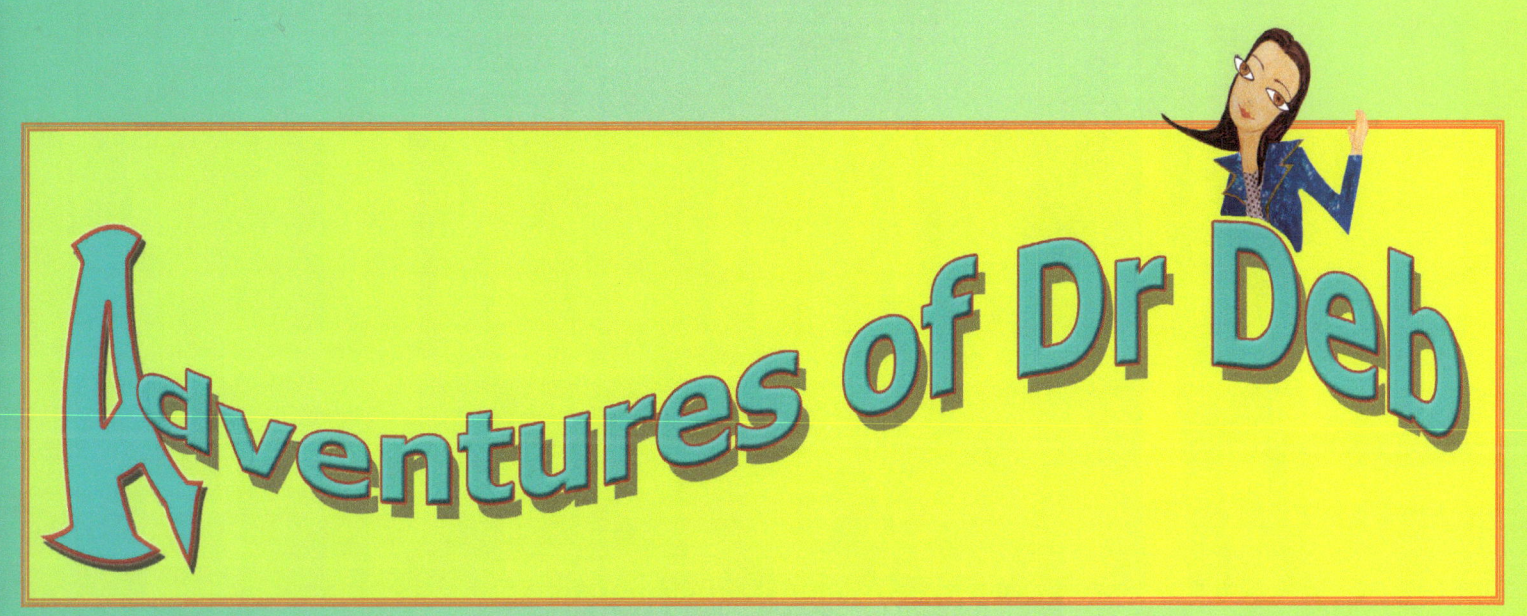

Adventures of Dr Deb

by Silvana Soriano & Debora Duro

Illustrated by Silvana Soriano

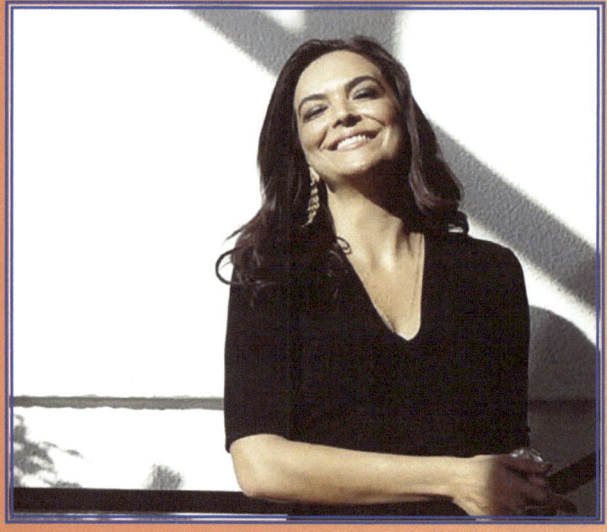

Dr. Debora Duro MD., MS.

Dr. Débora Duro is a physician born in São Jeronimo, Rio Grande do Sul, Brazil trained in Pediatric Gastroenterology, Hepatology and Nutrition at Boston Children's Hospital at Harvard Medical School. She is currently the director of the Pediatric Gastroenterology, Hepatology and Nutrition Program at the Broward Health, Fort Lauderdale, Florida, USA. Dr. Deb Duro earned a Master's Degree in Science and Dietetics from Florida International University. Her passion is to educate parents and families about the importance of teaching children to eat healthy meals since early childhood.
www.icangastroenterogy.com

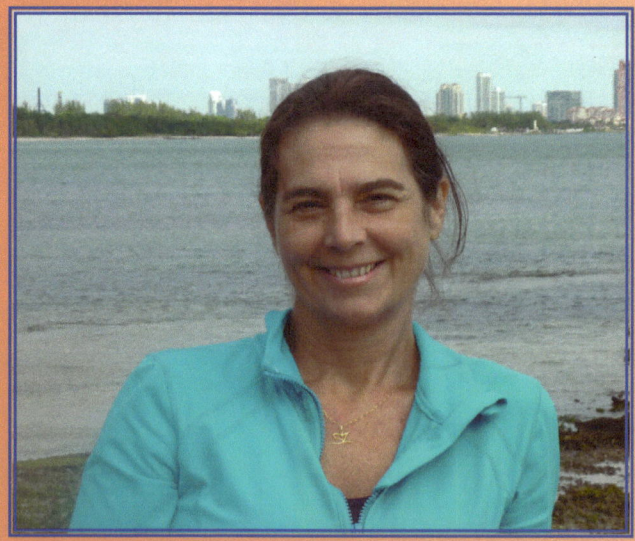

Silvana Soriano

Silvana Soriano was born in the city of Rio de Janeiro, Brazil. Visual artist, illustrator and arts teacher, she has always been surrounded by images. She received a bachelor's degree in Art Education at the Bennett University and, for many years, studied at the School of Visual Arts, Parque Lage, Rio deJaneiro. After moving to the United States in 2007, she started illustrating children`s books, as well as a collection of books on Modern Art for children. Currently, she also works as a Visual Arts teacher for the City of Miami`s public school system.

www.silvanasoriano.com

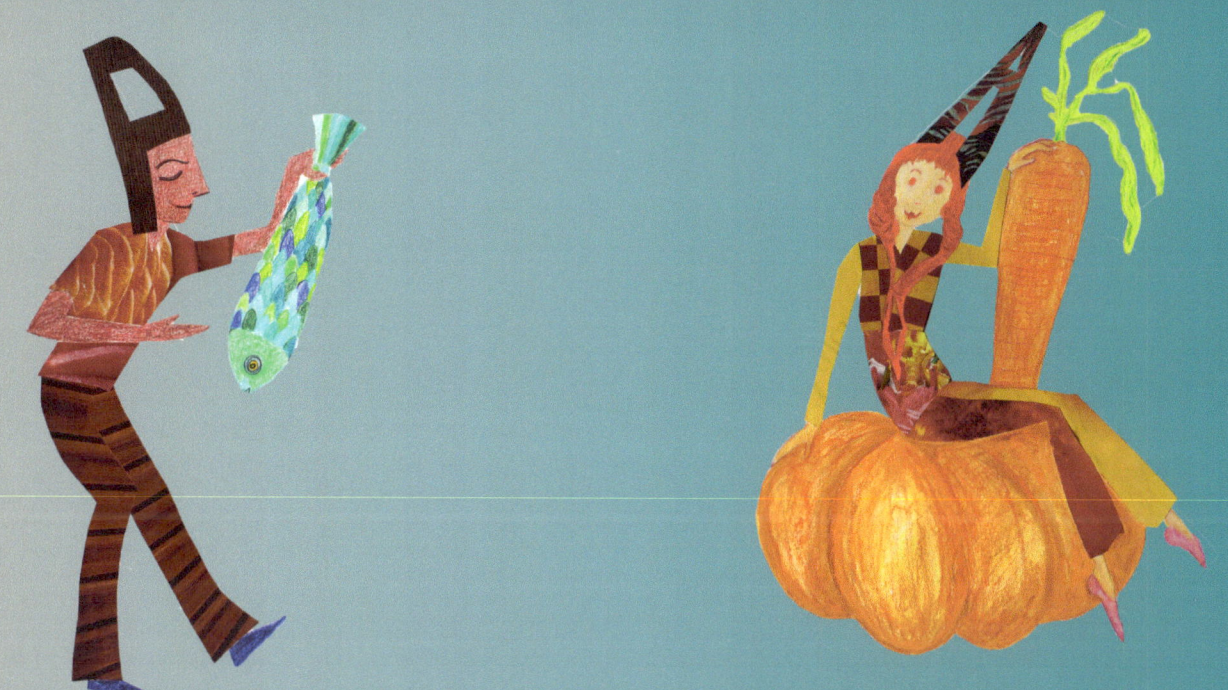

This book is dedicated to all kids in special for
Ana Ceci Duro de Araujo, Julio and Sofia Soriano.

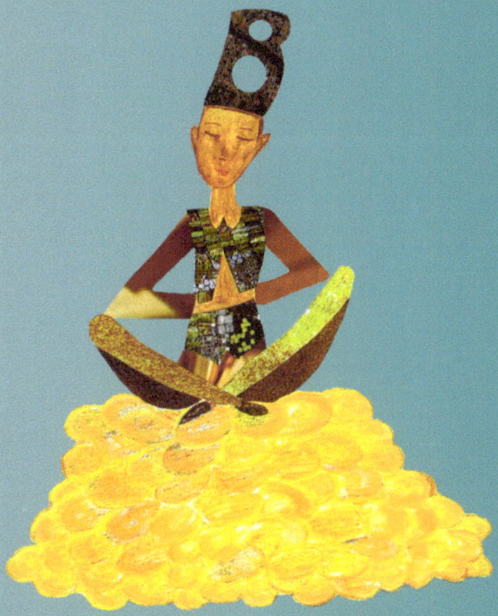

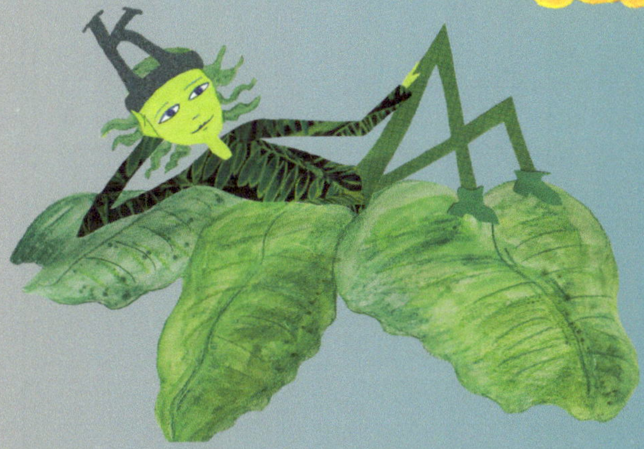

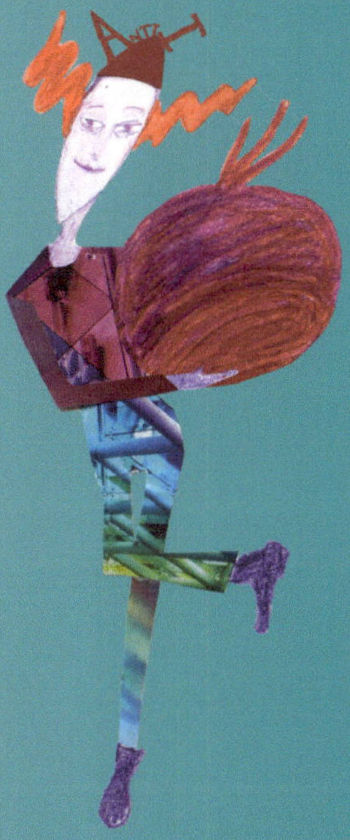

Sitting at the dining table, Ana cries out:

"I don't like vegetables! I don't want them!"

Aunt Deb smiles at the tantrums, and proposes:

"Ana, you did not even try them... Let's make a deal: I will tell you a story while you try some beet to see how it tastes."

Although a little wary, Ana accepted the suggestion, because she LOVED stories.

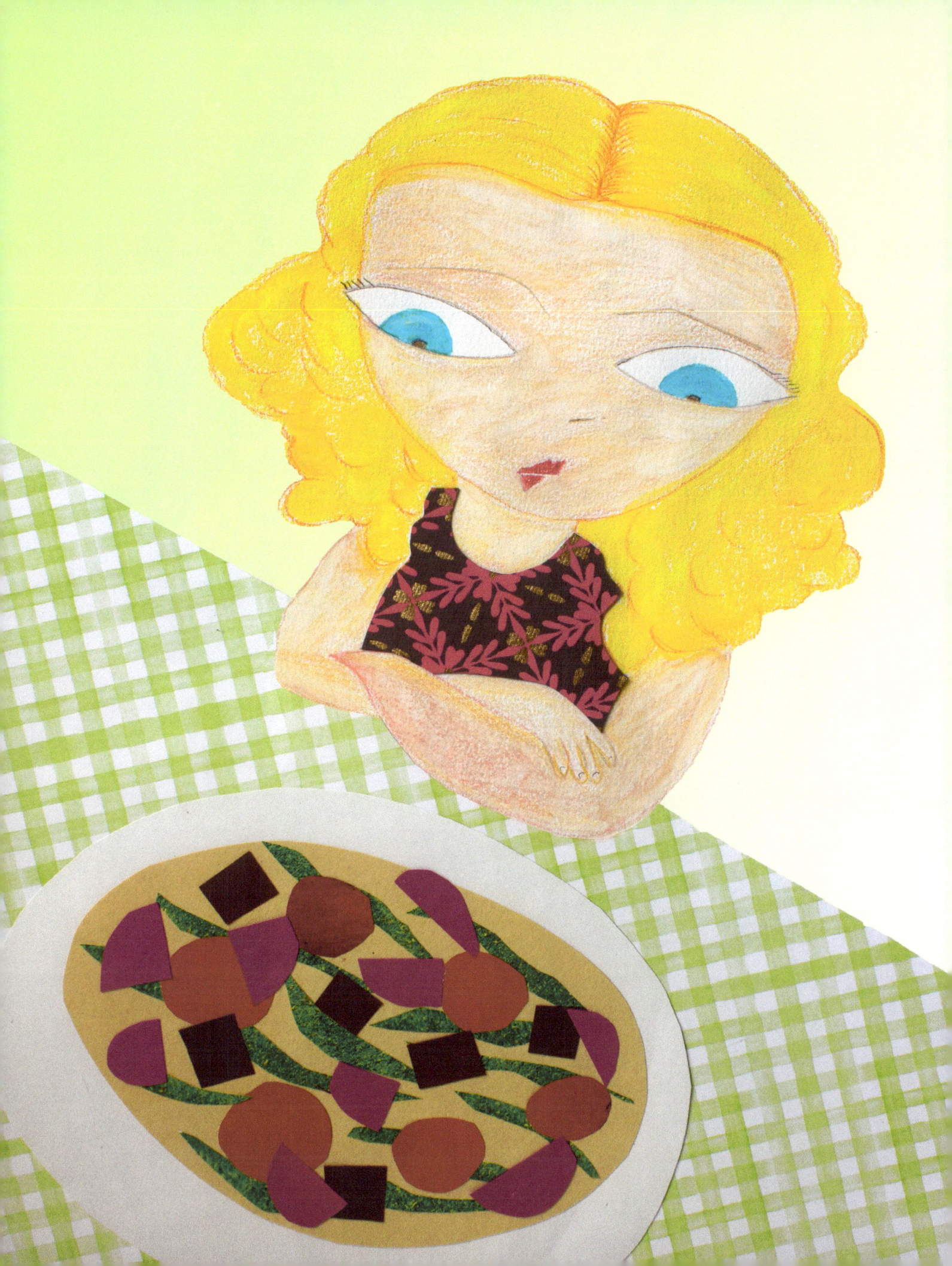

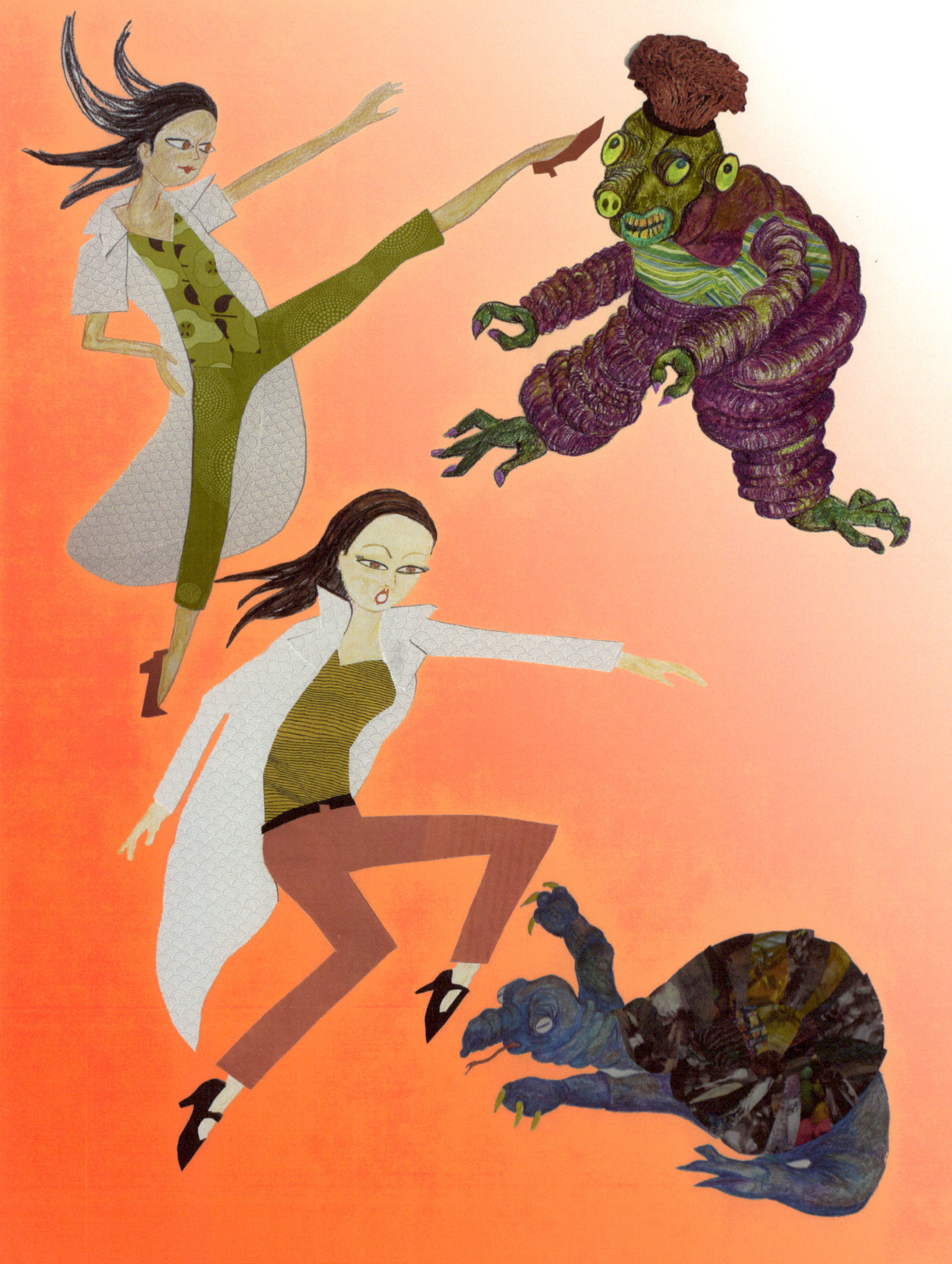

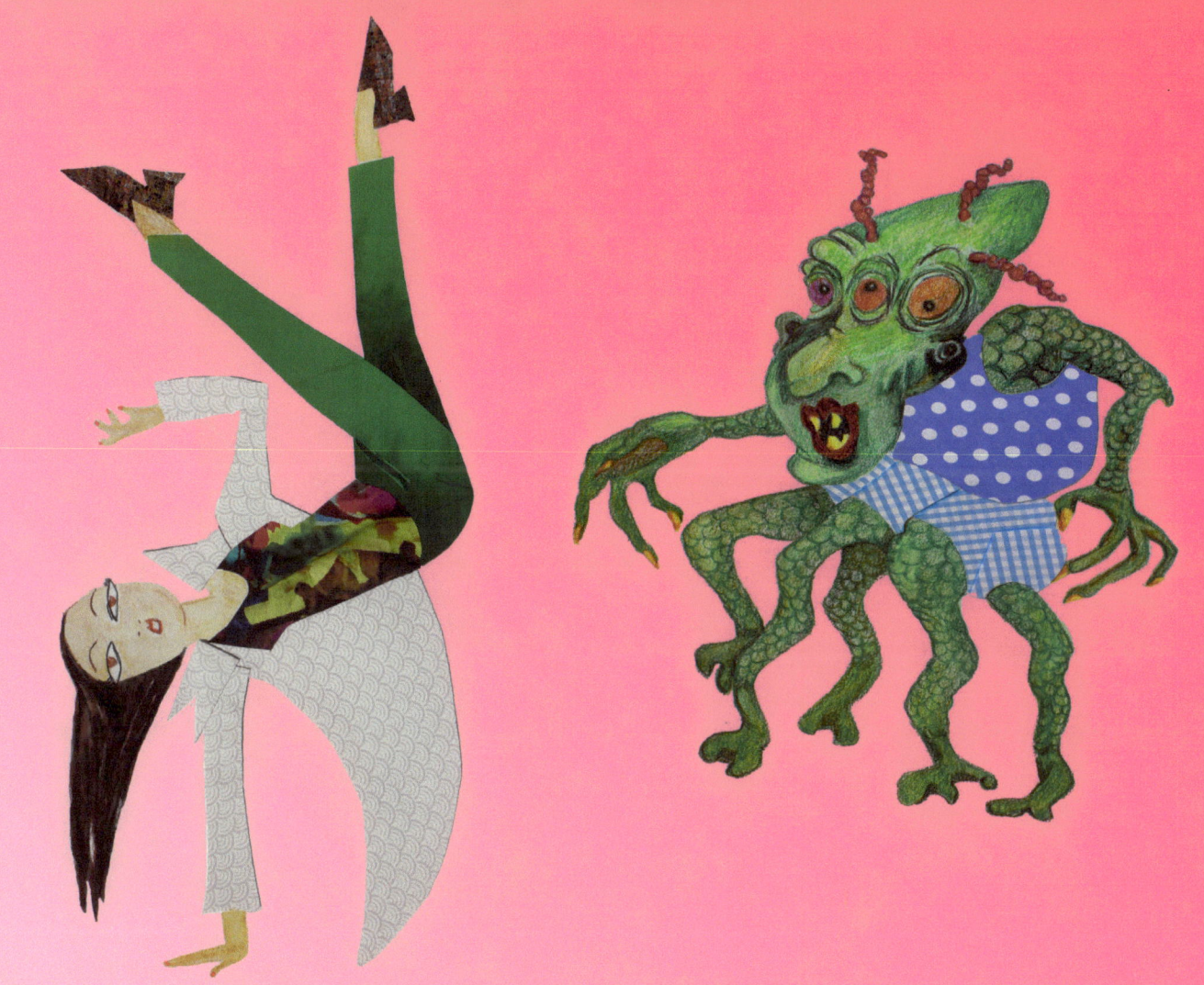

Once upon a time there was a doctor, Dr. Deb, who worked on a large hospital. She loved to take care of children. She was strong, courageous and always ready to fight against diseases. She struggled against the monster of tummy ache, or against the super snail of motion sickness, or even against the terrible goblin of hard stool. And she always overcame them all. There was, however, a very powerful enemy. Her name was Sadie, the witch of sadness. With this one, the battle was hard.

One day, a very weak boy came in with a terrible tummy ache! Dr. Deb began to fight it! She transformed that belly monster into a tiny mouse, that fled, scared. When she went out to assist another boy, she saw tears running down his face. She froze in fear! At that moment, Dr. Deb saw a dark shadow moving over the wall. The shadow was making a noise that scared everyone nearby. Using its arms, which seemed like tentacles, it grasped what was ahead.

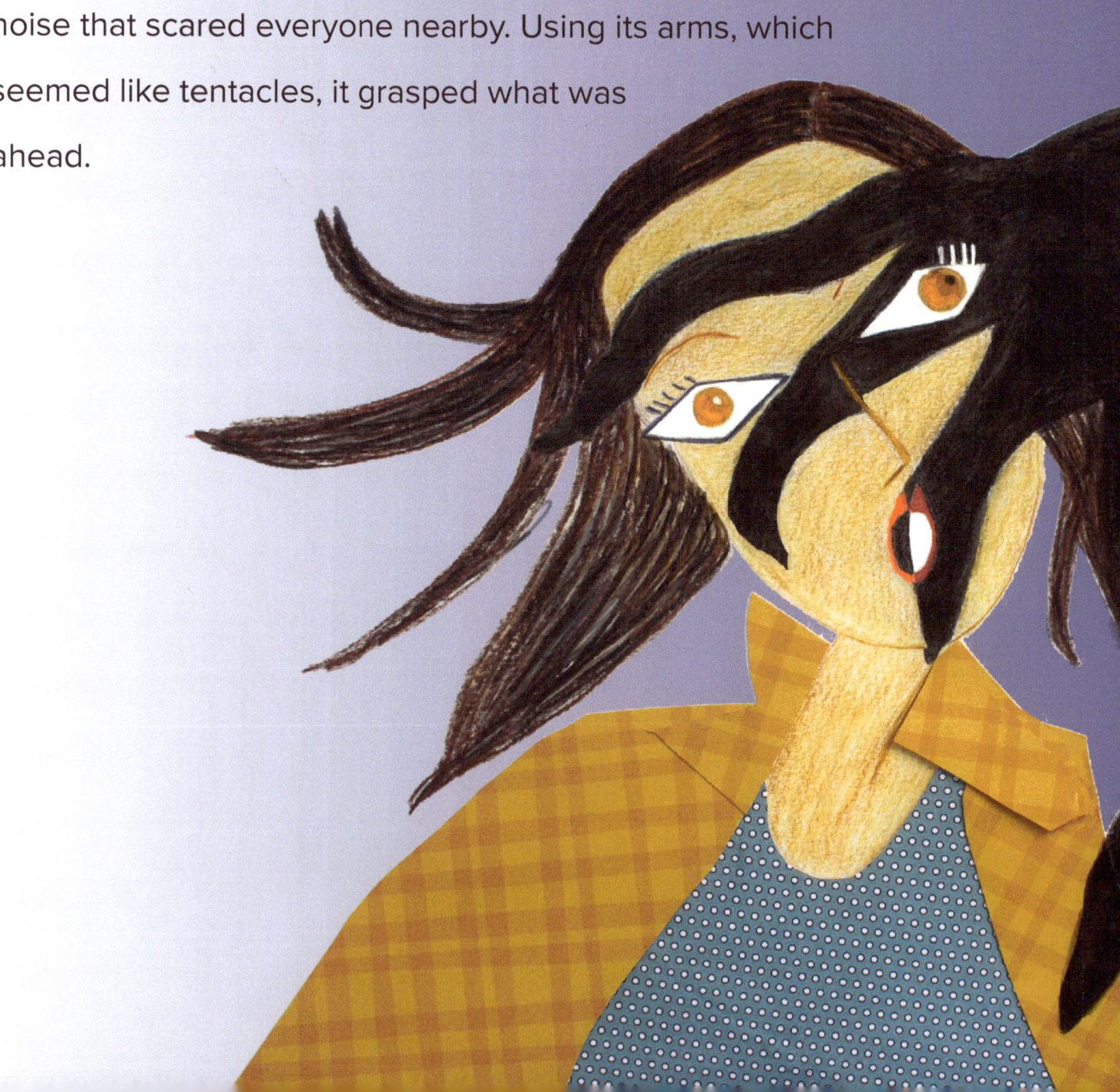

It was the most feared, the more grotesque, and powerful witch Sadie! However hard she tried, Dr. Deb could not find a way to fight her. And the witch was getting bigger and bigger, increasingly ugly, increasingly alarming!

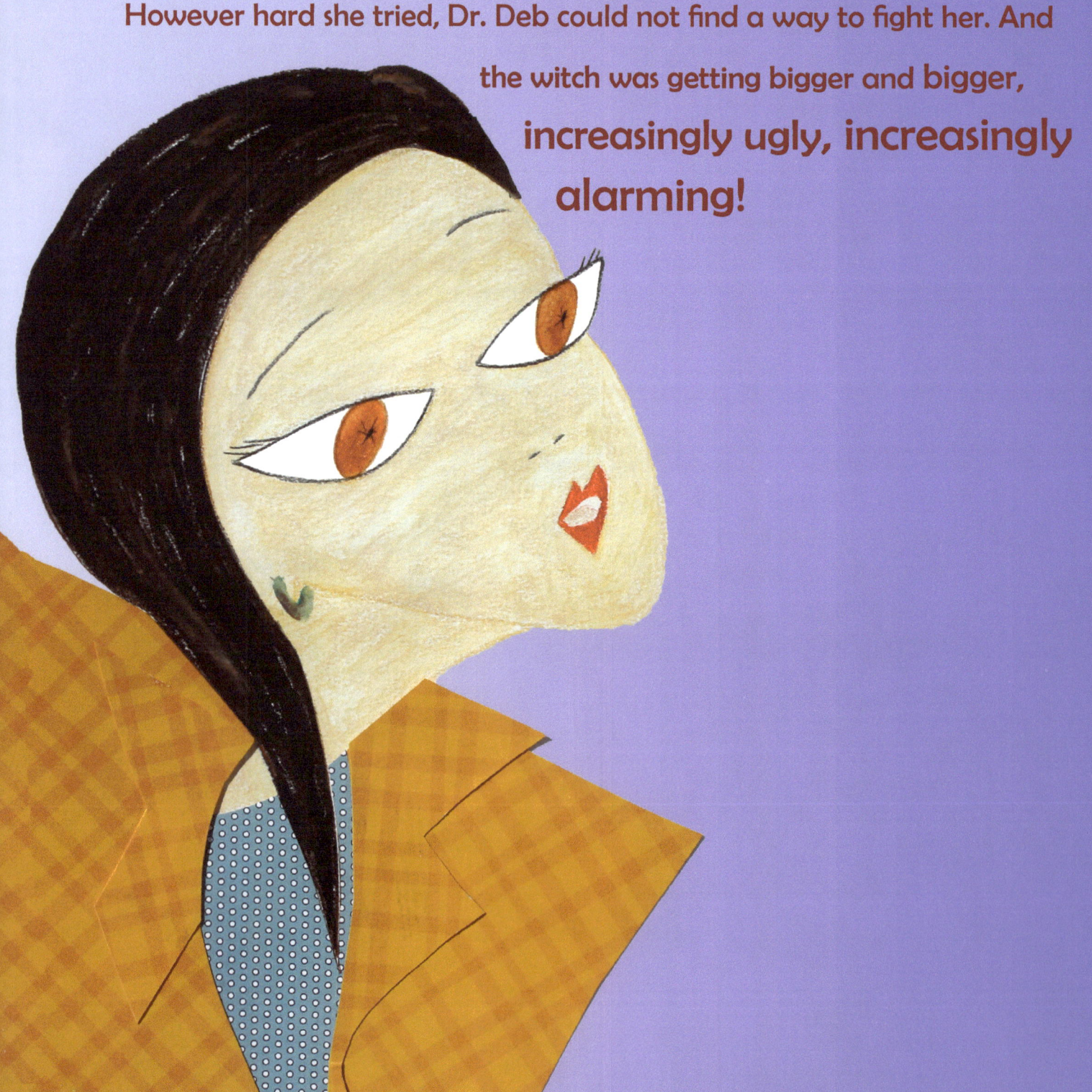

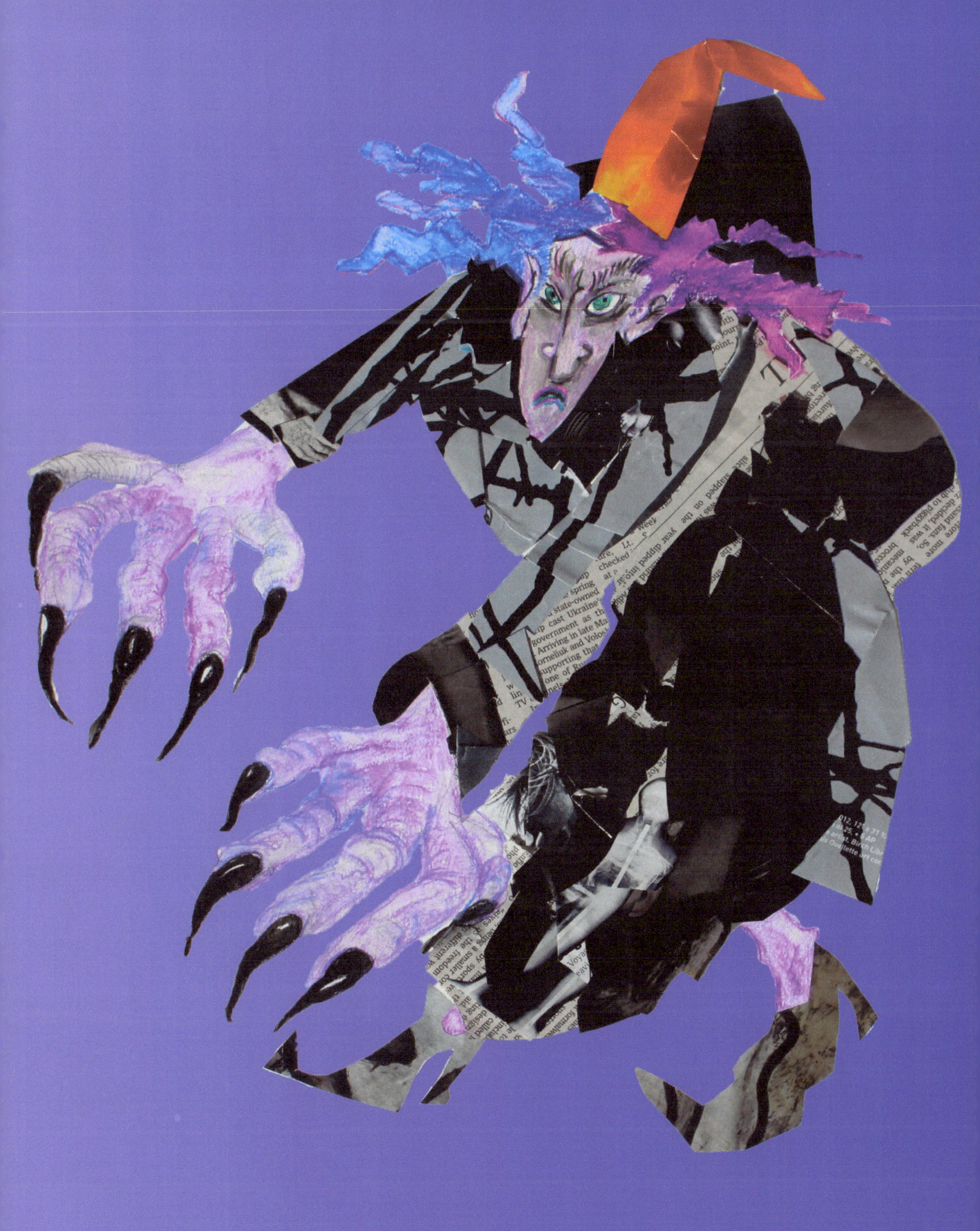

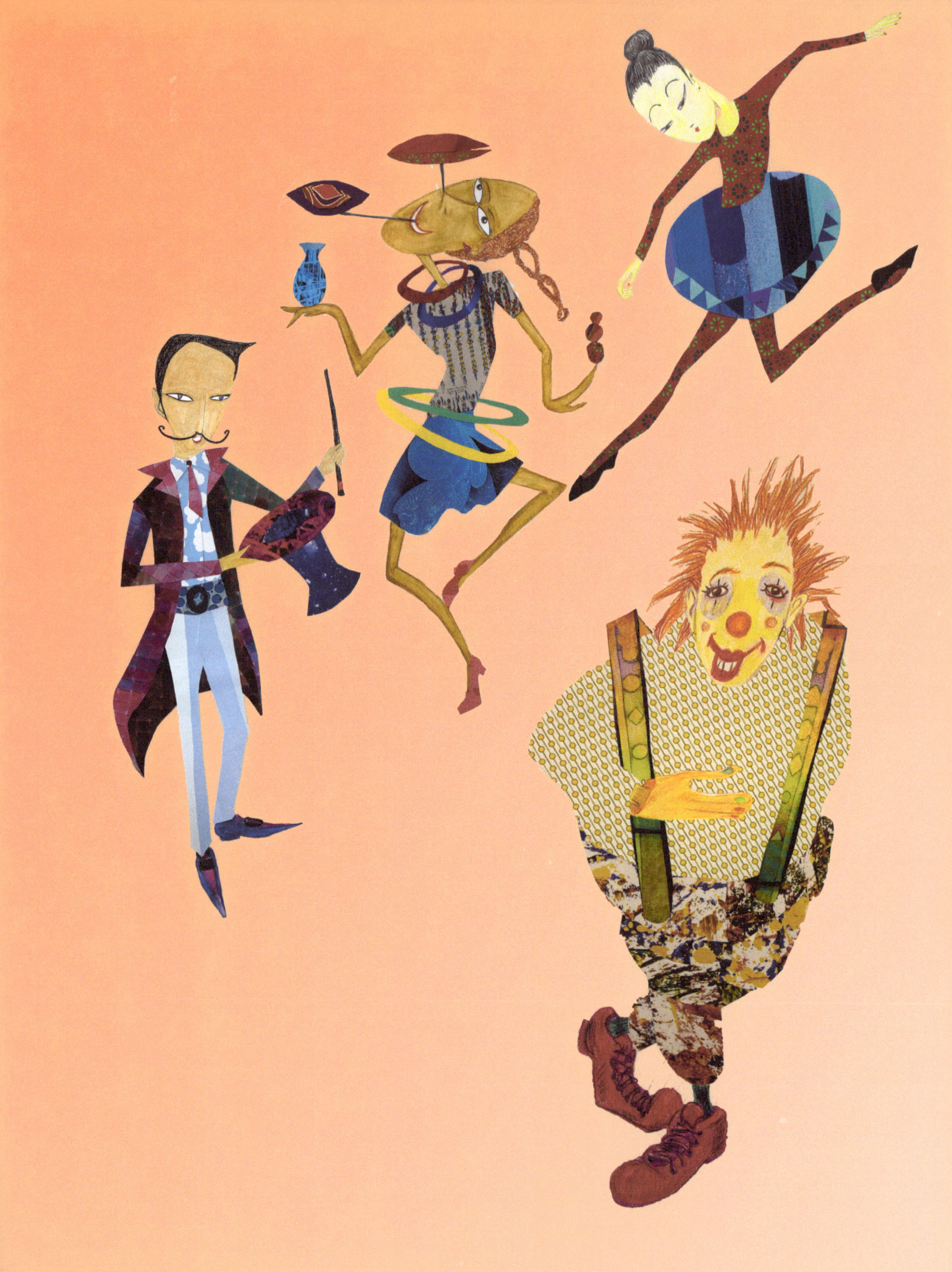

At that moment, a bunch of noisy and colorful people entered the bedroom! A clown, a magician, a juggler and a ballerina. They were all laughing and singing. Ignoring the awful witch, they greeted the boy and the doctor, clowning around and joking. And, believe it or not, the witch, as if by magic, disappeared! Dr. Deb was amazed!

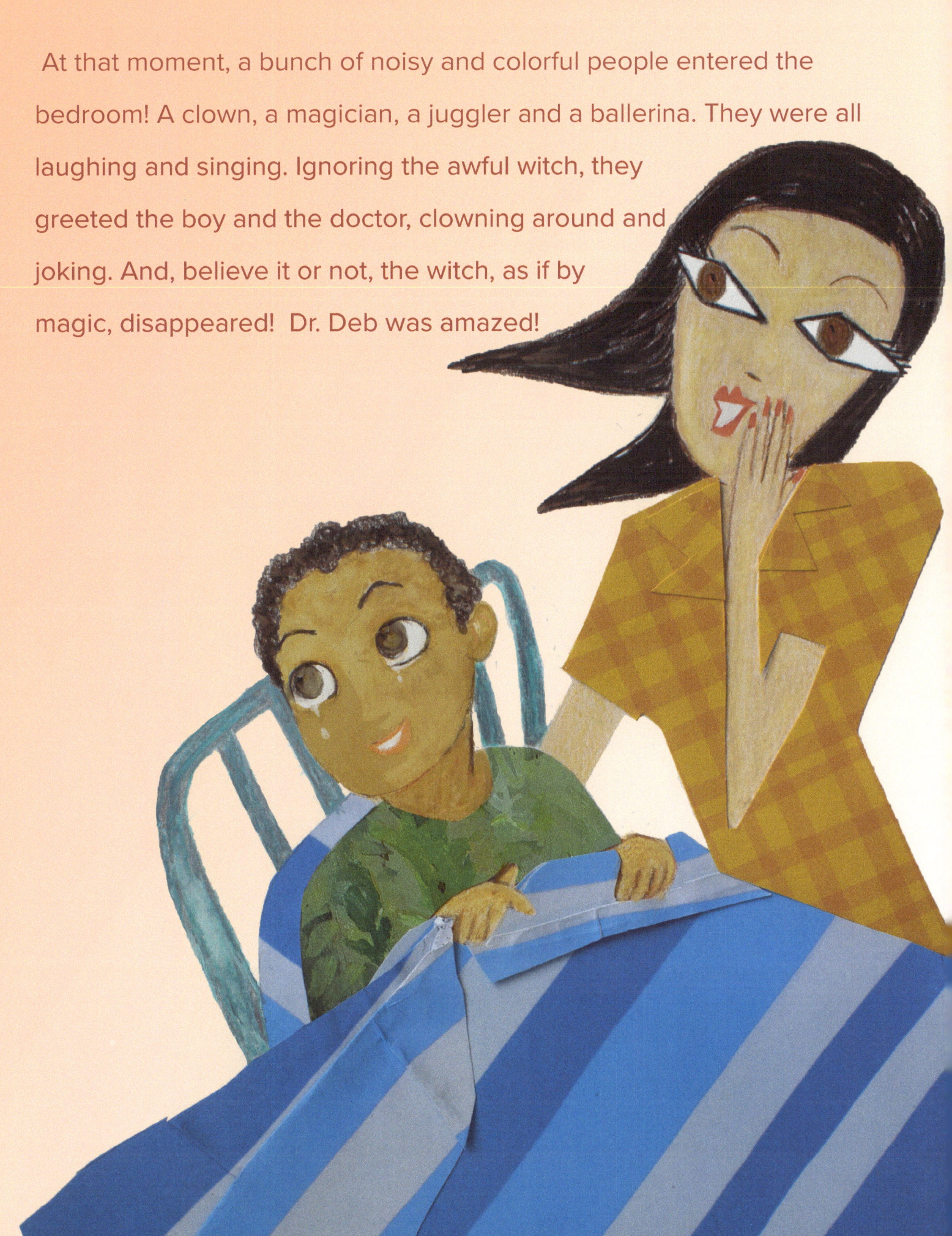

The clown cleared his throat and said:

"We are from the circus of Joy, and Joy is our medicine!"

"Wow, I need this formula right away!" said Dr. Deb.

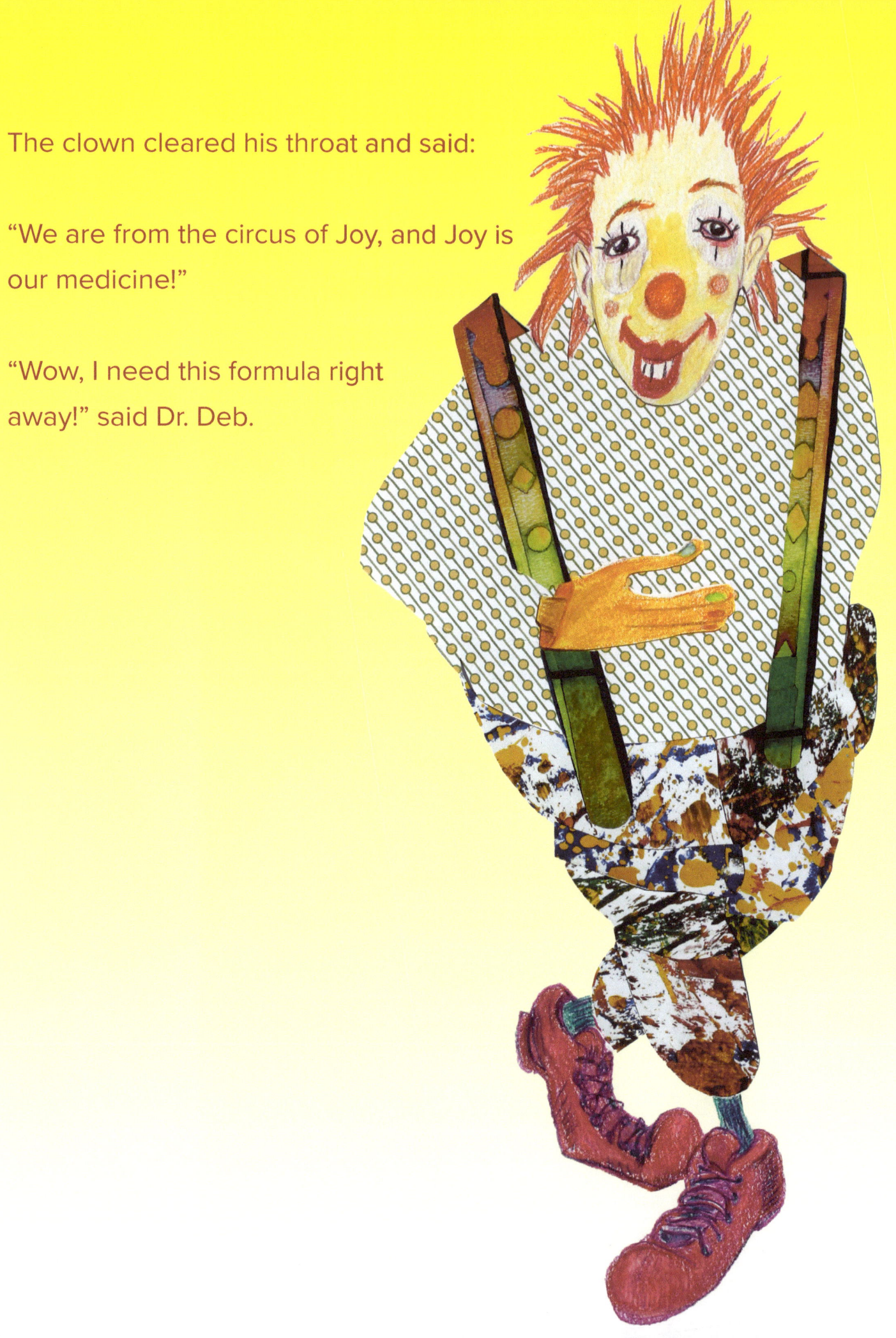

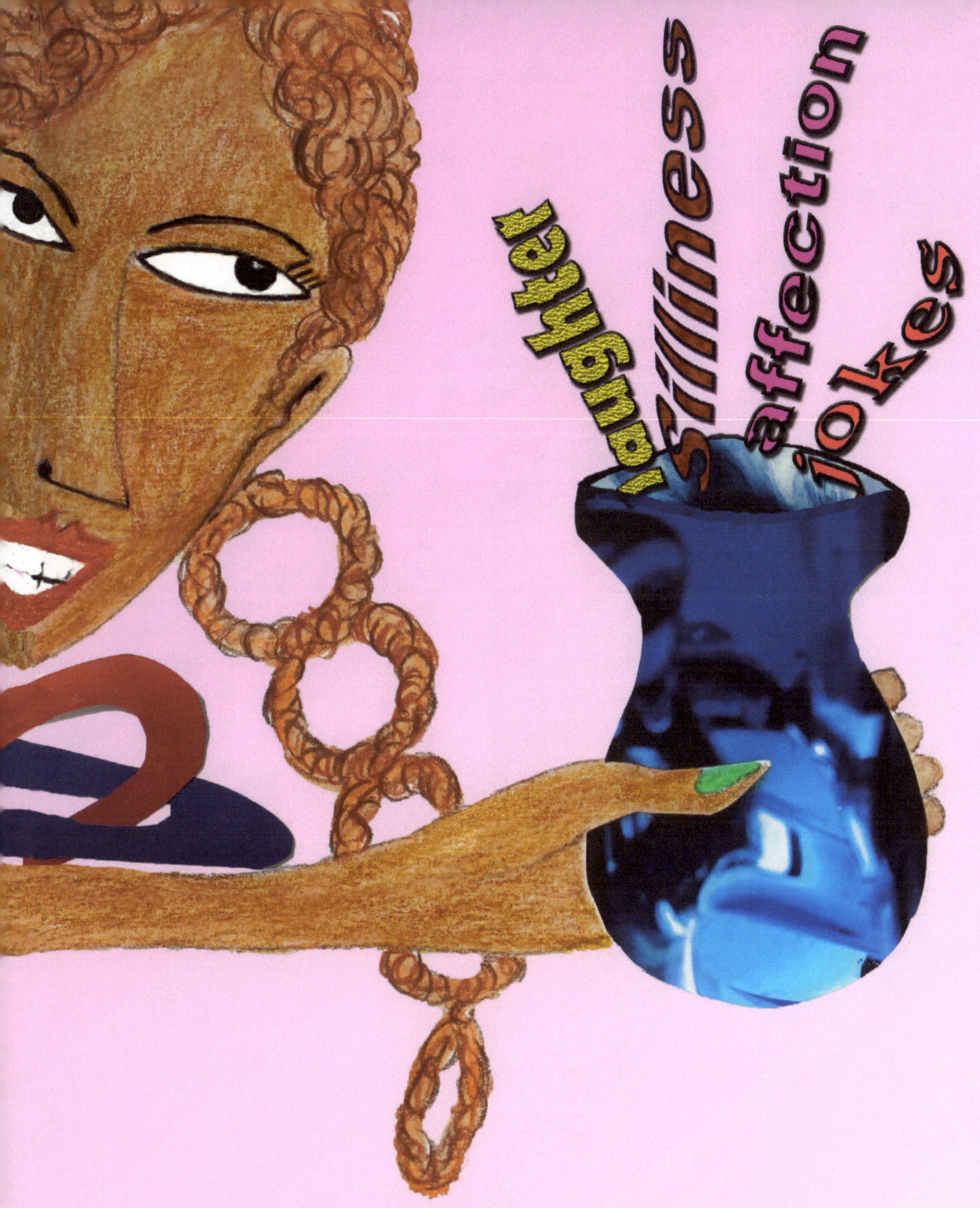

laughter

silliness

affection

jokes

The juggler, bringing a strange bottle, added:

"It's a very simple formula: 1 pinch of clowning, 2 tablespoons of laughs, 1 glass of silliness and, finally, 1 handful of hugs. Mix everything up and the medicine is ready!"

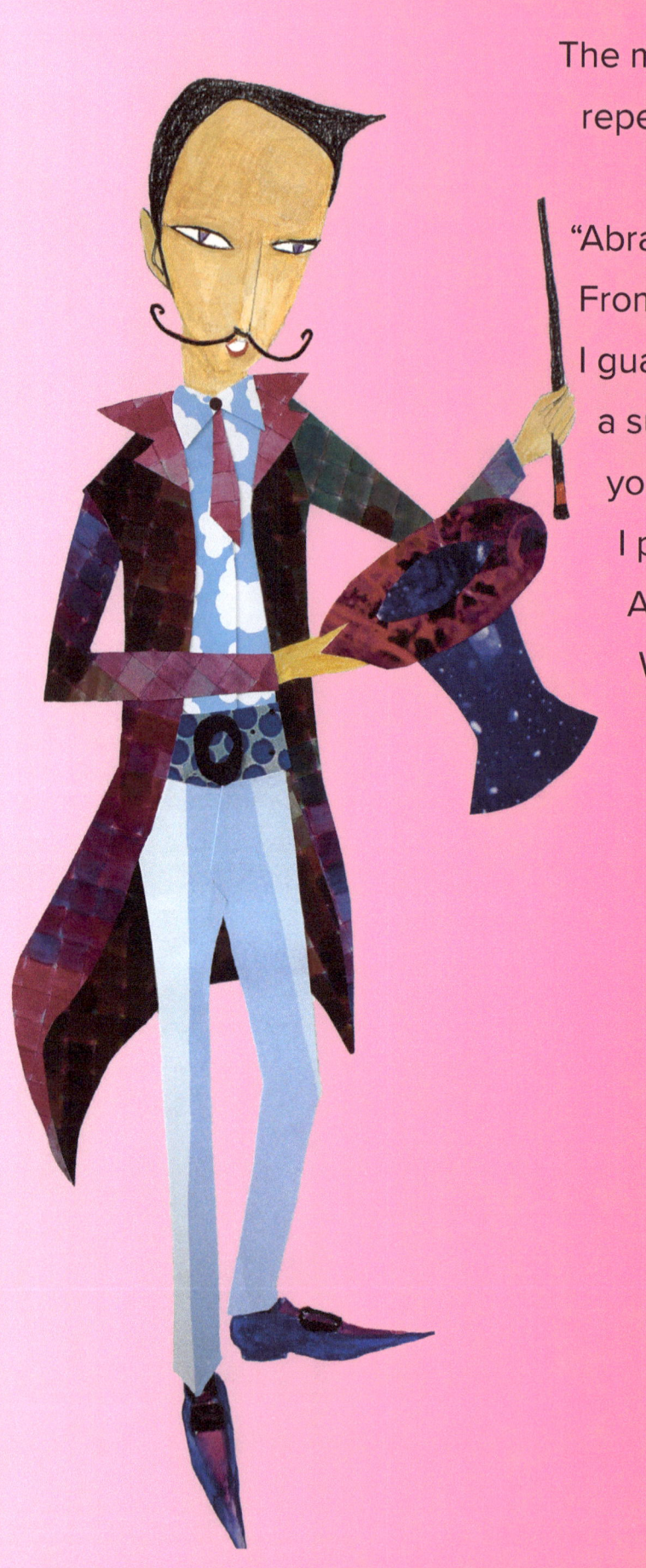

The magician, addressing the doctor,
repeated:

"Abracadabra,
From the top hat,
I guarantee,
a surprise will appear,
you just wait and see,
I promise to do my best!
And what comes next?
With these eyeglasses
you can read from the inside out.
It is the way, beyond any doubt,
to take care of these kids!"

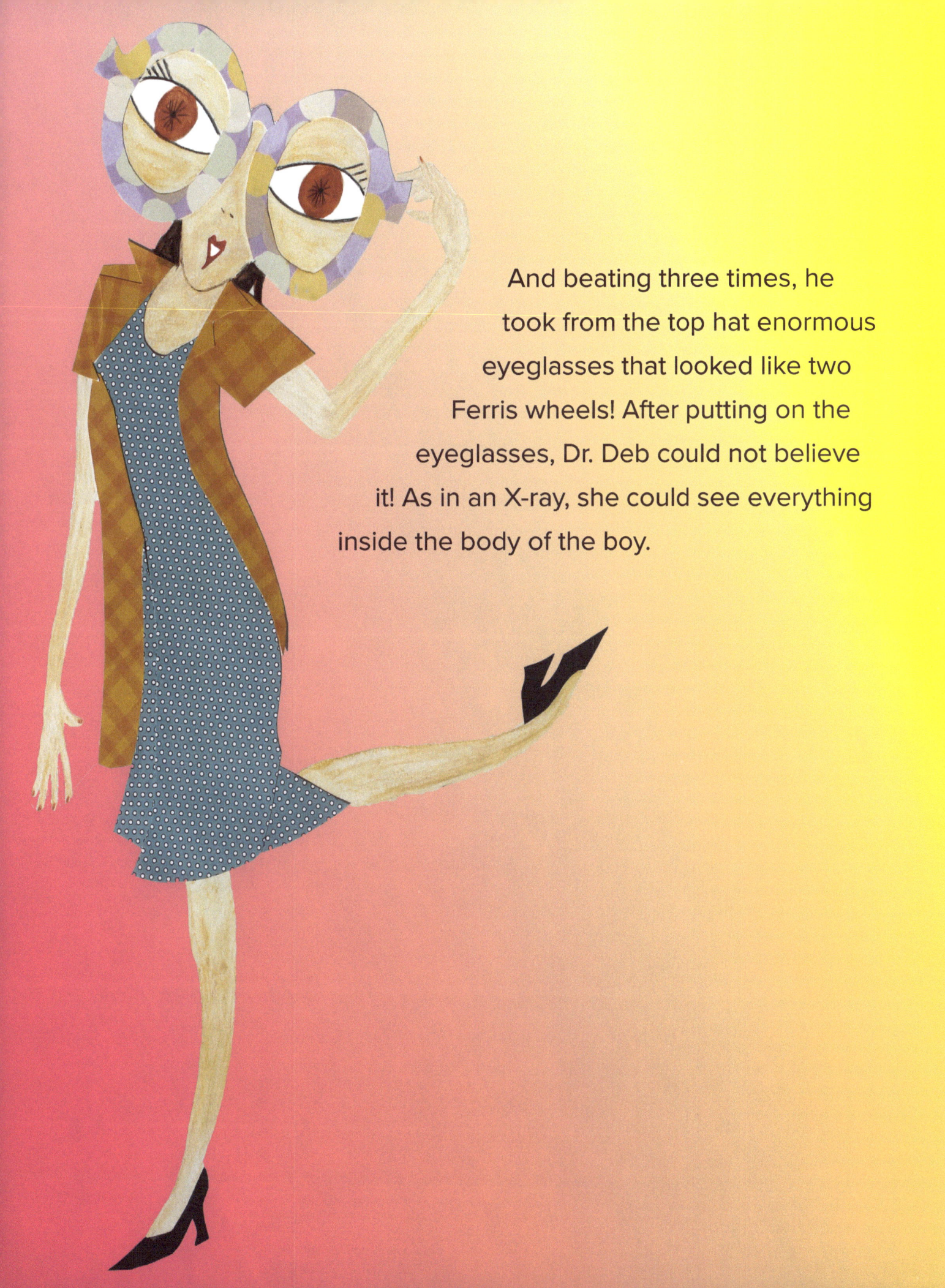

And beating three times, he
took from the top hat enormous
eyeglasses that looked like two
Ferris wheels! After putting on the
eyeglasses, Dr. Deb could not believe
it! As in an X-ray, she could see everything
inside the body of the boy.

Since then, the hospital has completely changed! Everything became colorful and cheerful. The children were not sad anymore. Monsters were not able to hide. Using the magic eyeglasses, Dr. Deb could find them in seconds! With the invisible power of joy and her magic eyeglasses, the doctor could help more children!

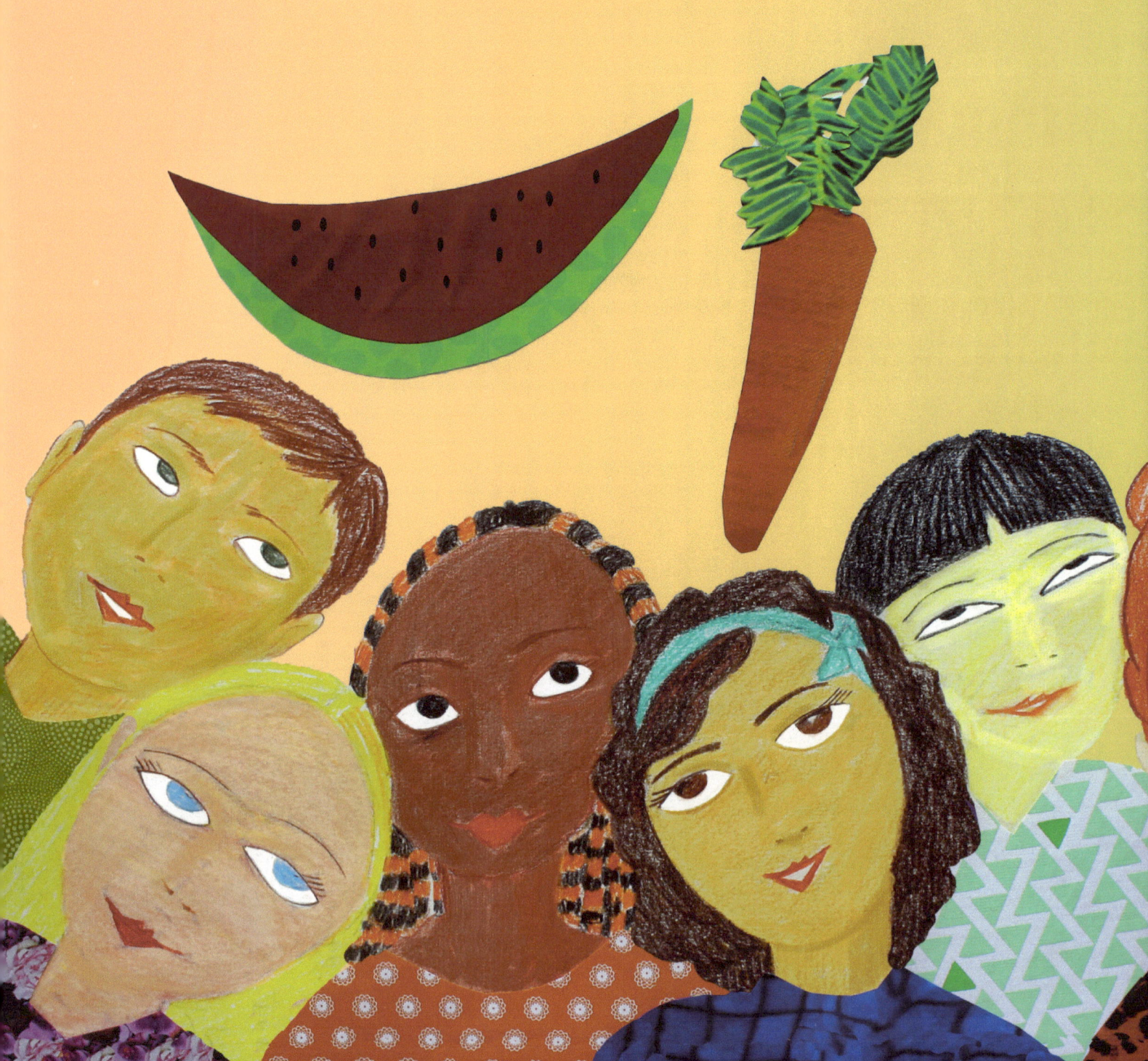

She took the circus of Joy everywhere she visited. Together they taught children about the delicious and colorful foods! Orange carrots, green broccoli, red watermelon and purple beets!

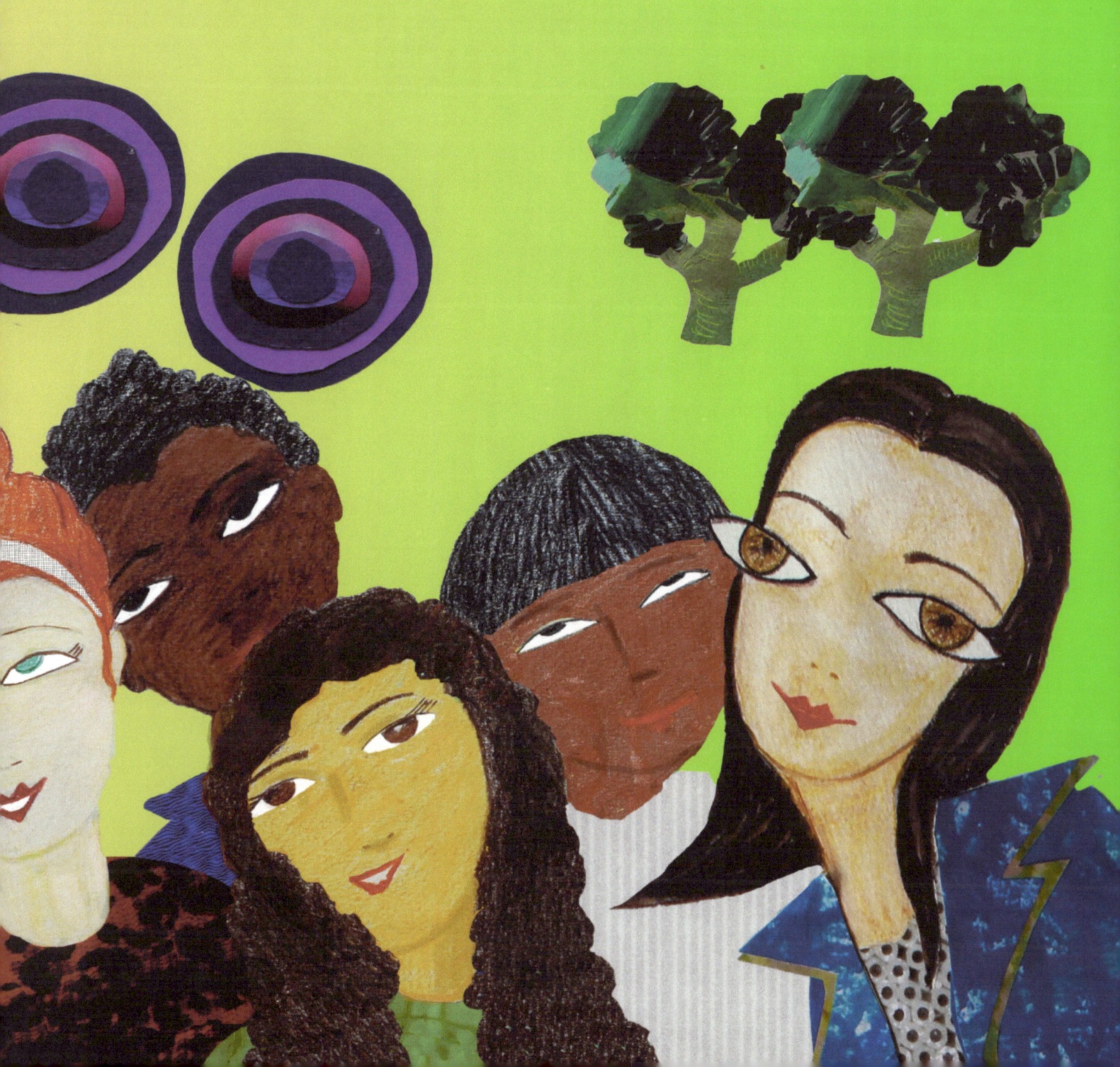

There was even a mathematical formula:

Color + Joy = Healthy Kids

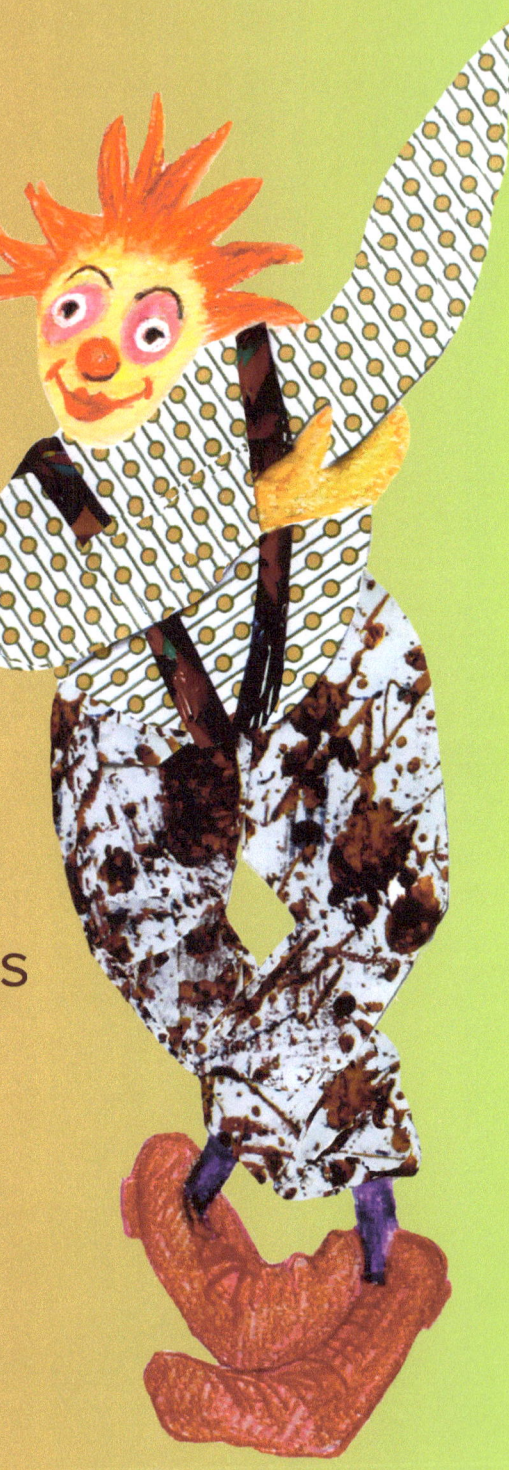

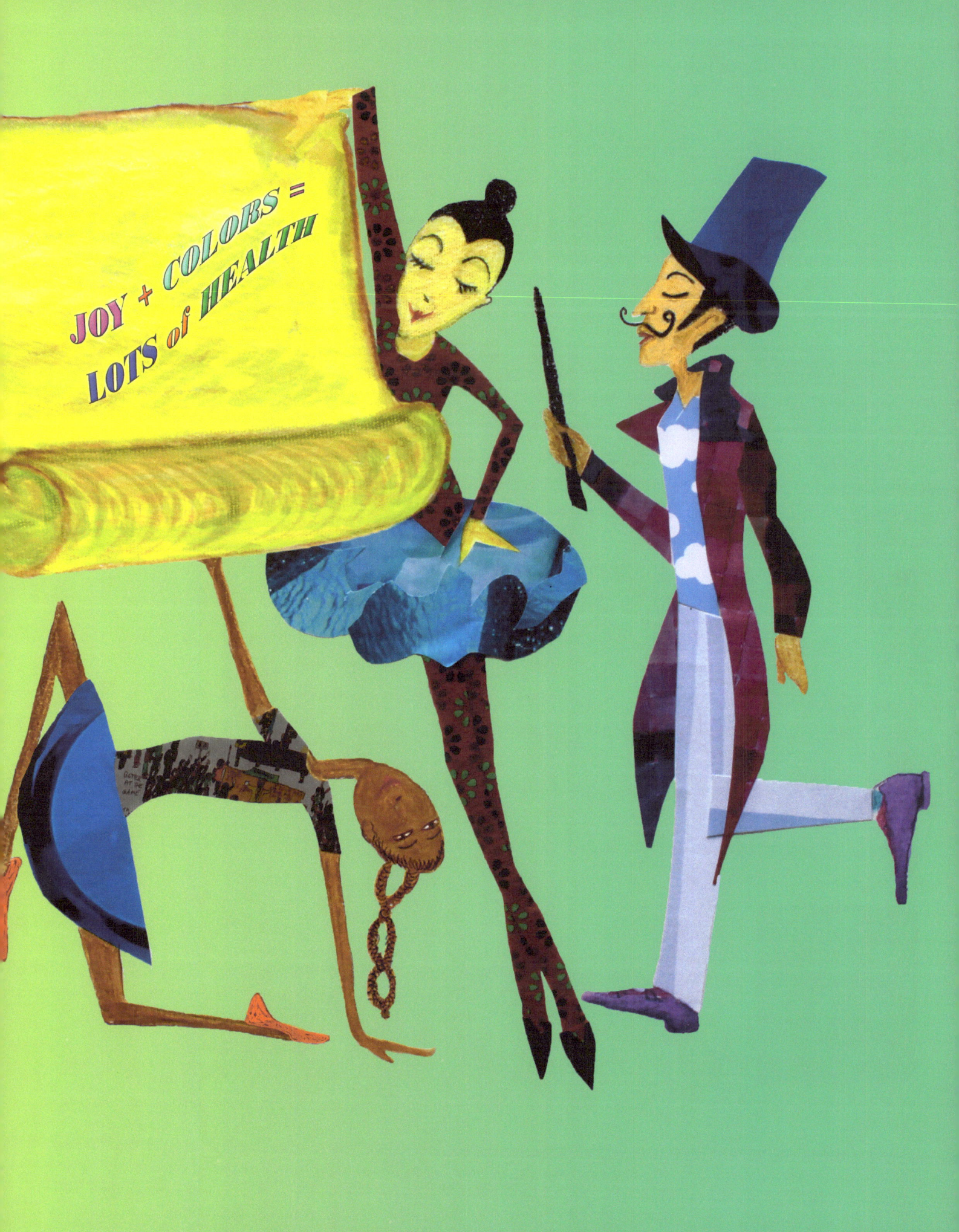

From her bag, Aunt Deb took her giant eyeglasses and handed them to Ana:

"Look at your plate with these eyeglasses and tell me what you see."

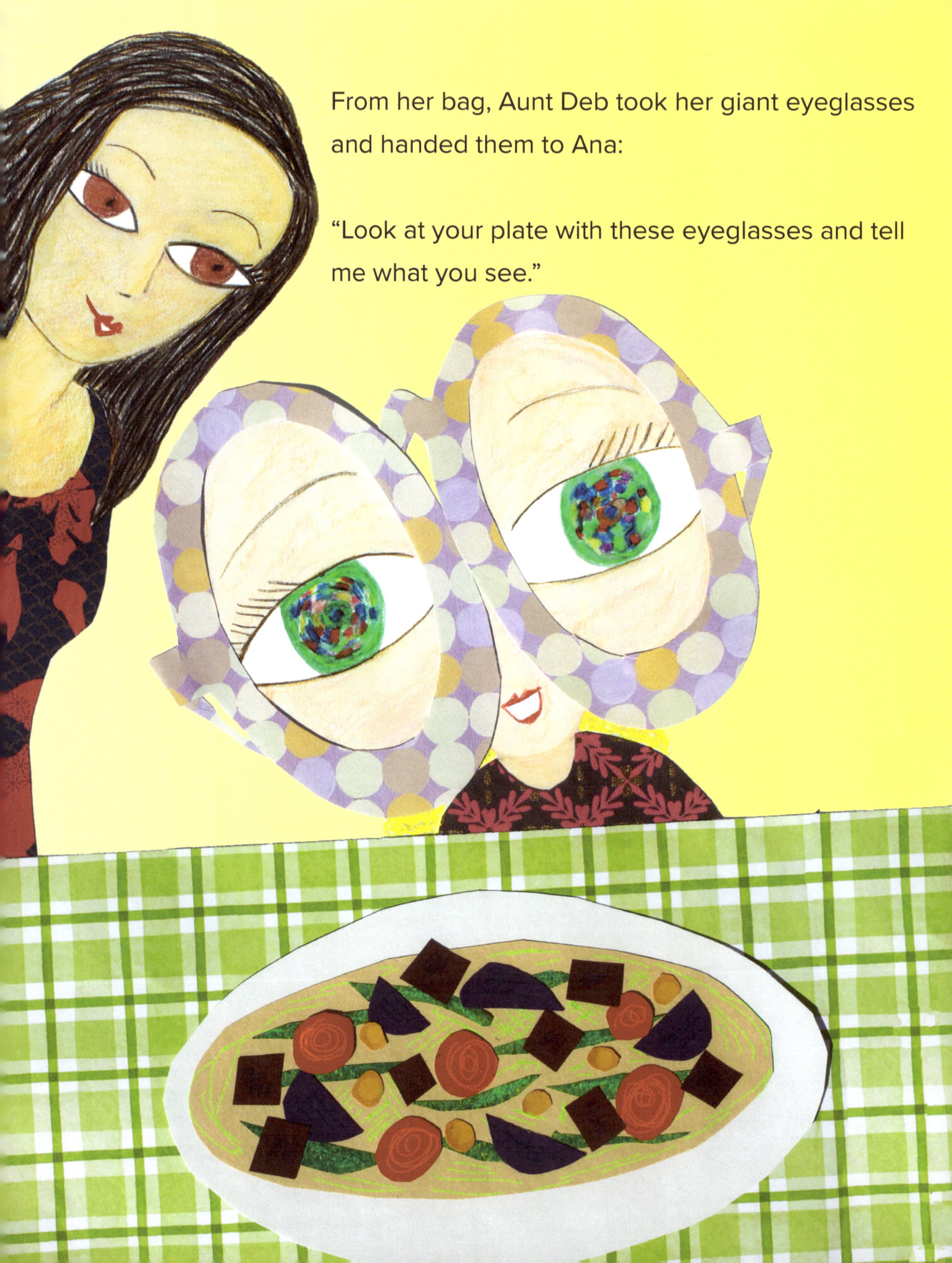

"Wow, what beautiful colors! Is this a rainbow soup?" Ana asked.

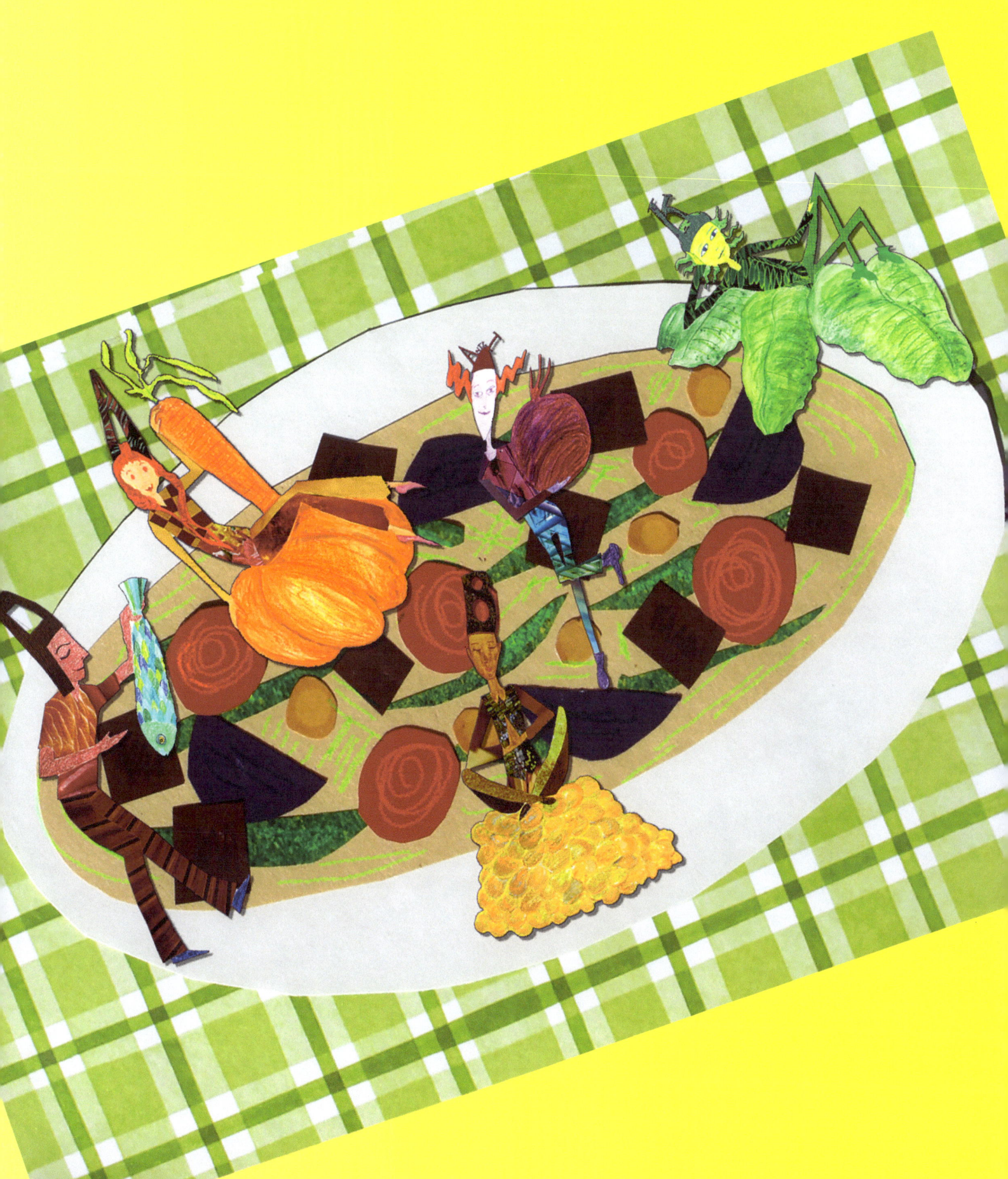

"Well, the purple color is the beet" Aunt Deb replied. "It has excellent anti-inflammatory properties and makes our eyes glitter. In pumpkins and carrots, the orange color is the vitamin A, which helps us to see better at night. Green kale leaves are full of vitamin K, which helps in blood coagulation. Golden lentils are rich in vitamin B, which makes the hair shine, and, finally, the brown chunks of meat, full of protein, make large and strong muscles."

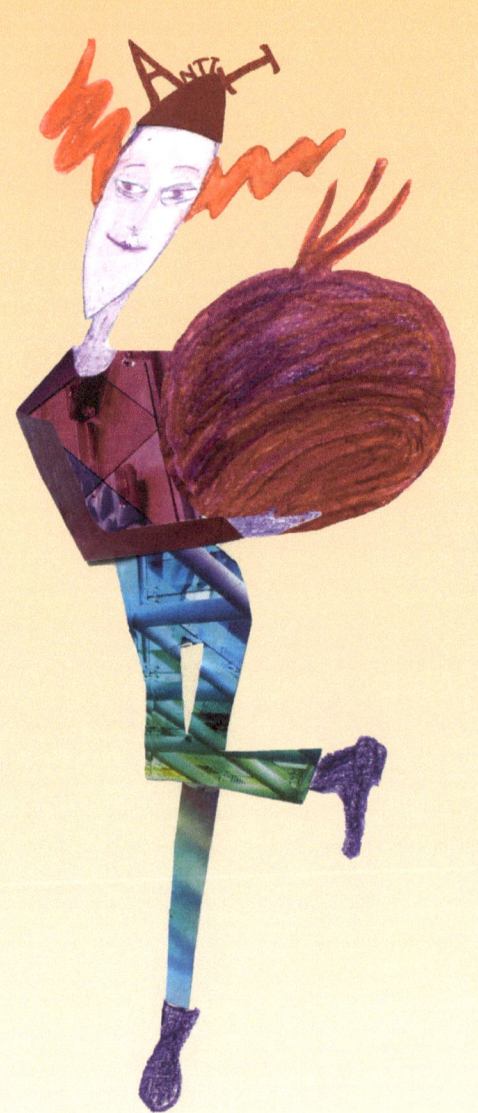

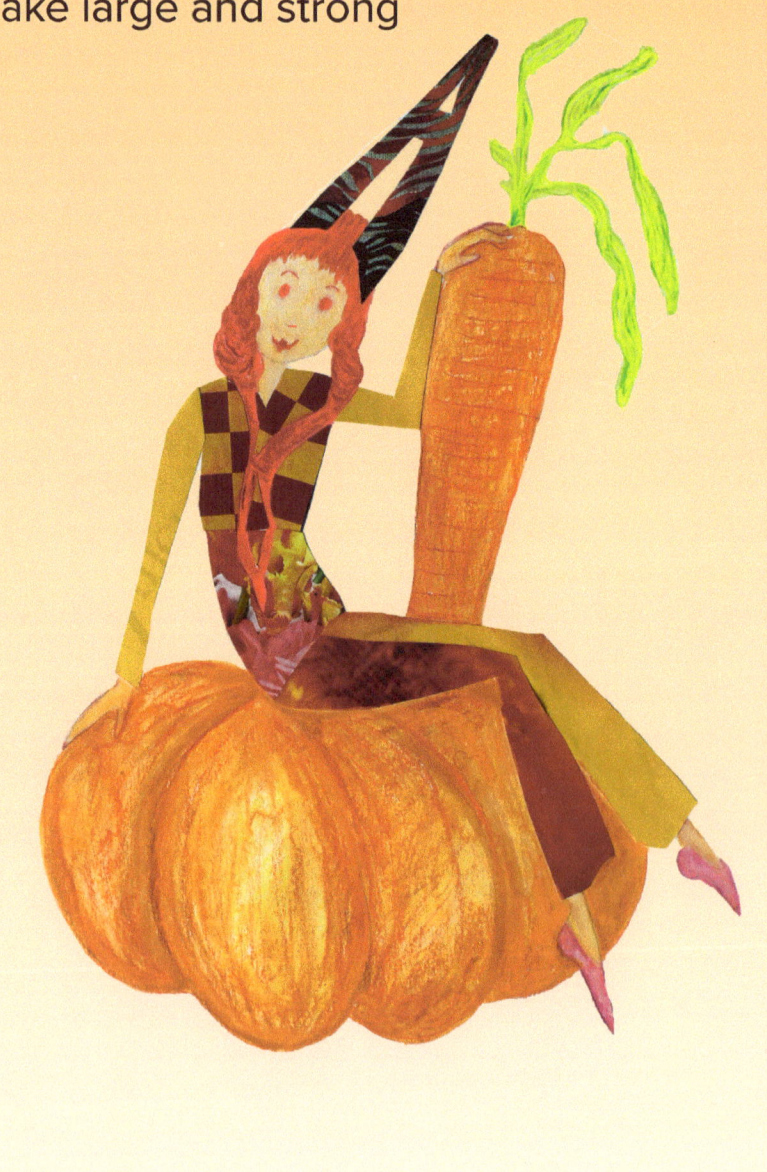

Ana was very curious. She tried everything that was on her plate. And she loved it!

As soon as she had finished, Aunt Deb suggested:

"Let's understand the story of foods from the beginning."

Ana nodded.

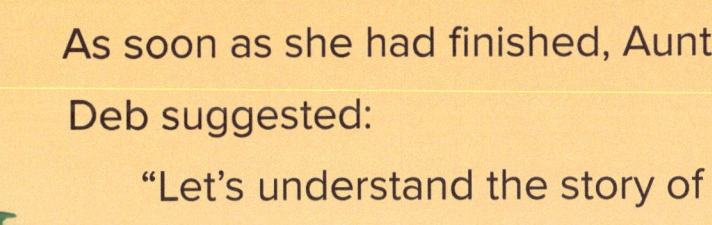

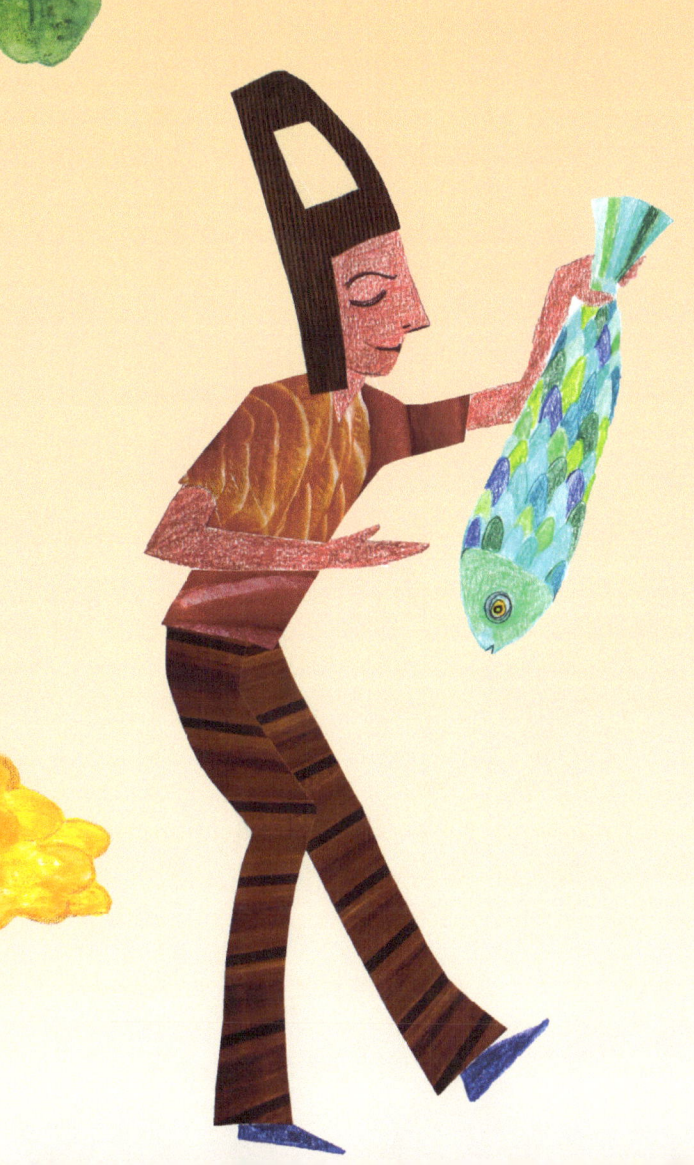

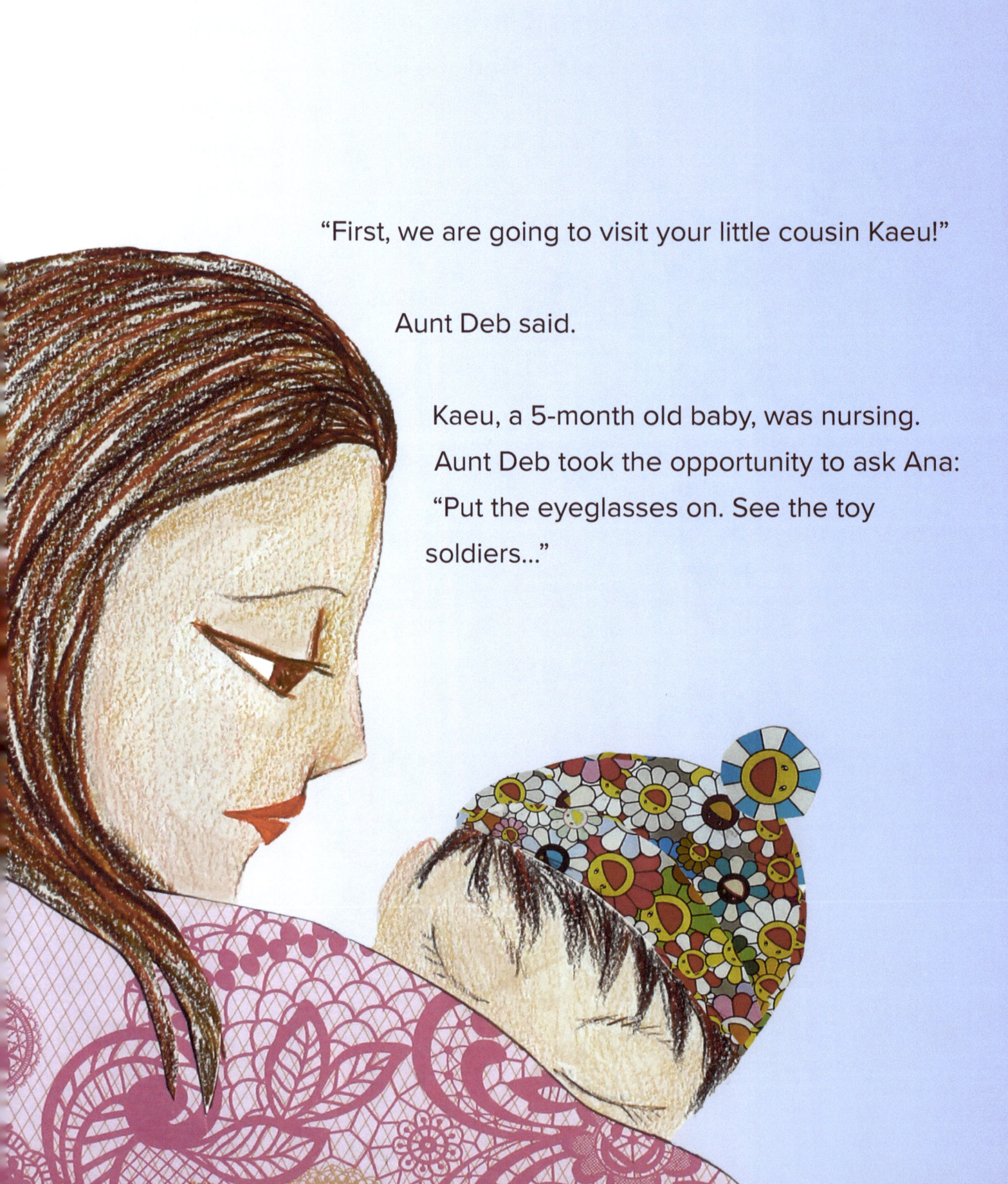

"First, we are going to visit your little cousin Kaeu!"

Aunt Deb said.

Kaeu, a 5-month old baby, was nursing.
Aunt Deb took the opportunity to ask Ana:
"Put the eyeglasses on. See the toy
soldiers..."

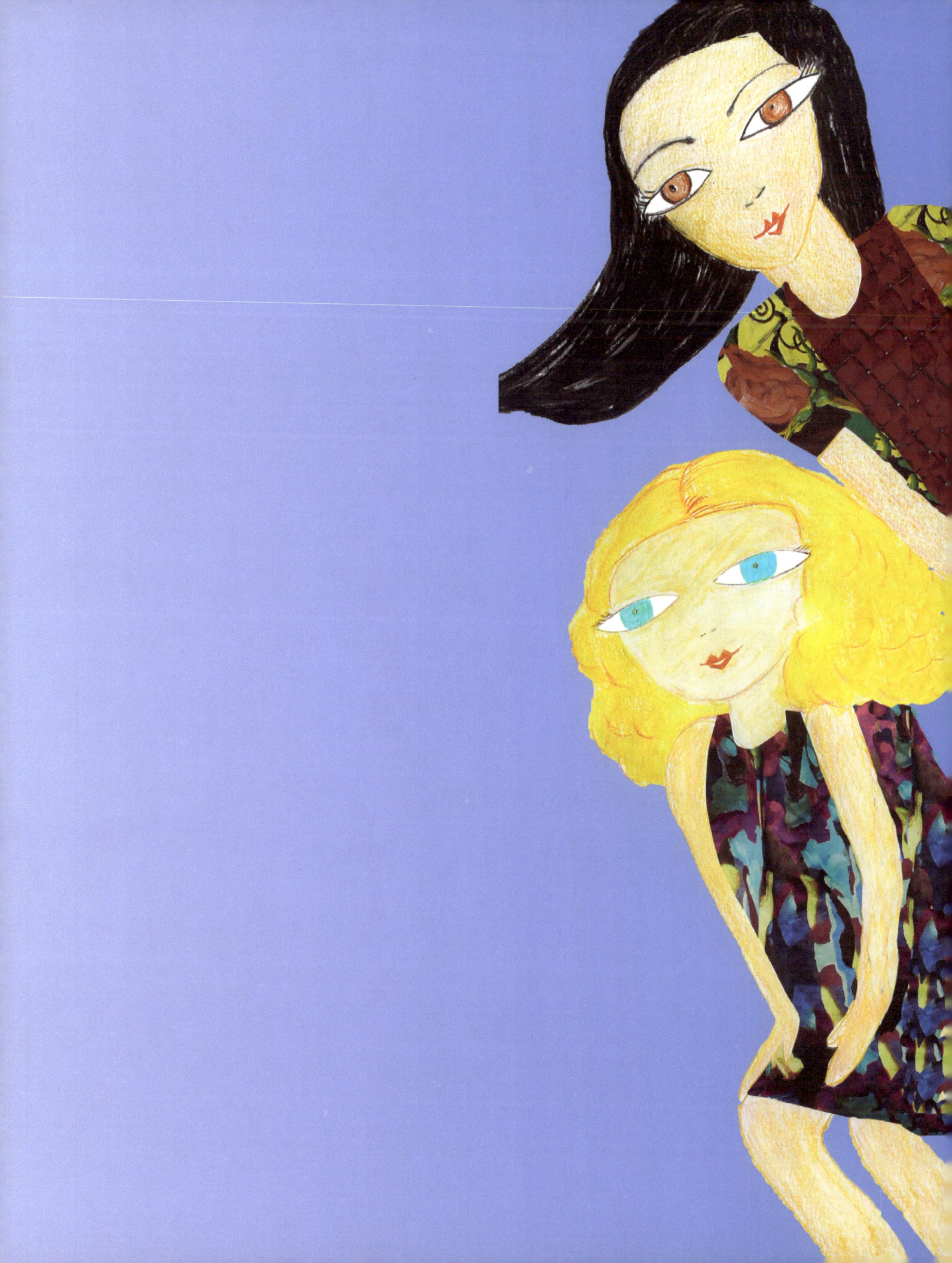

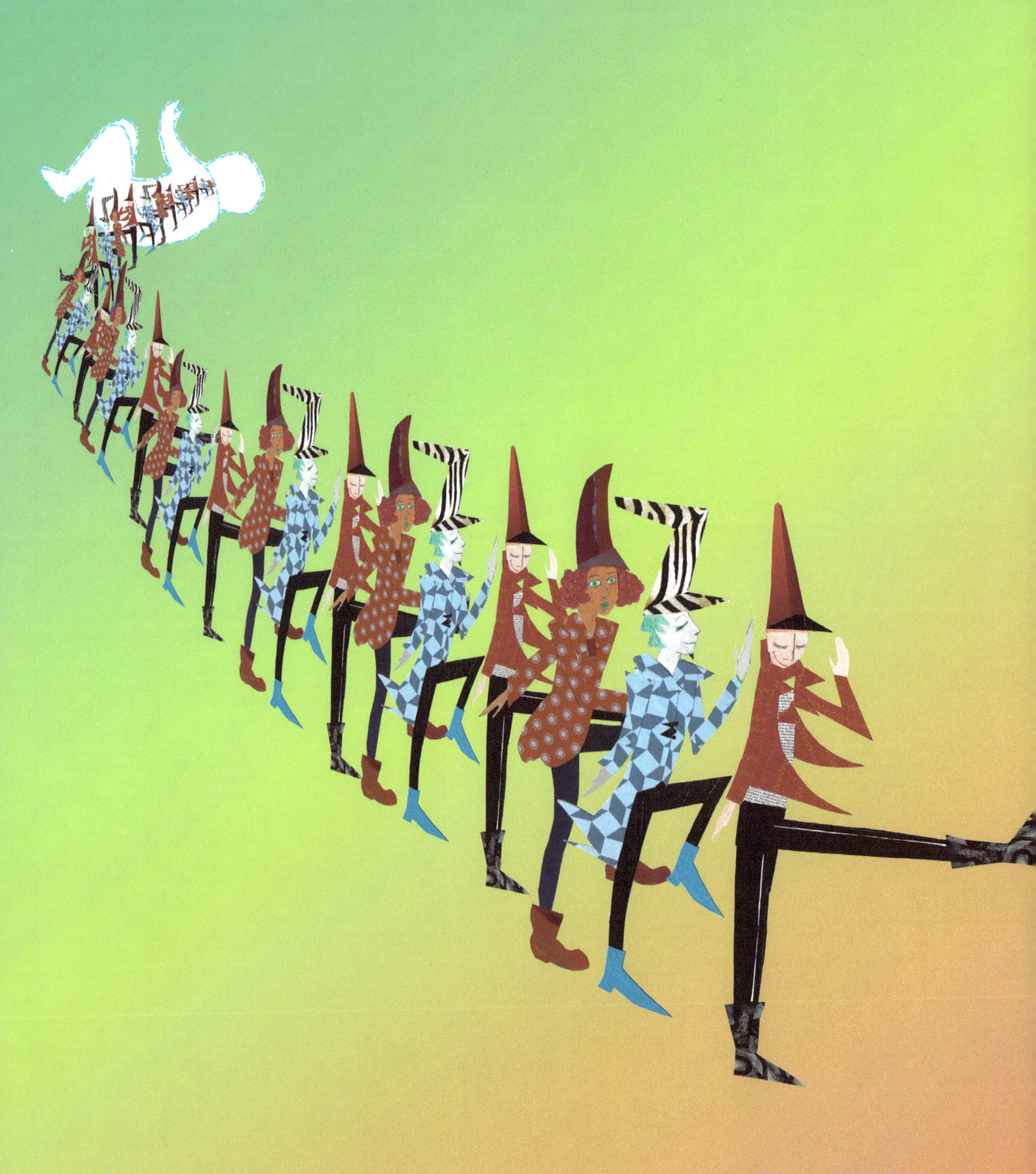

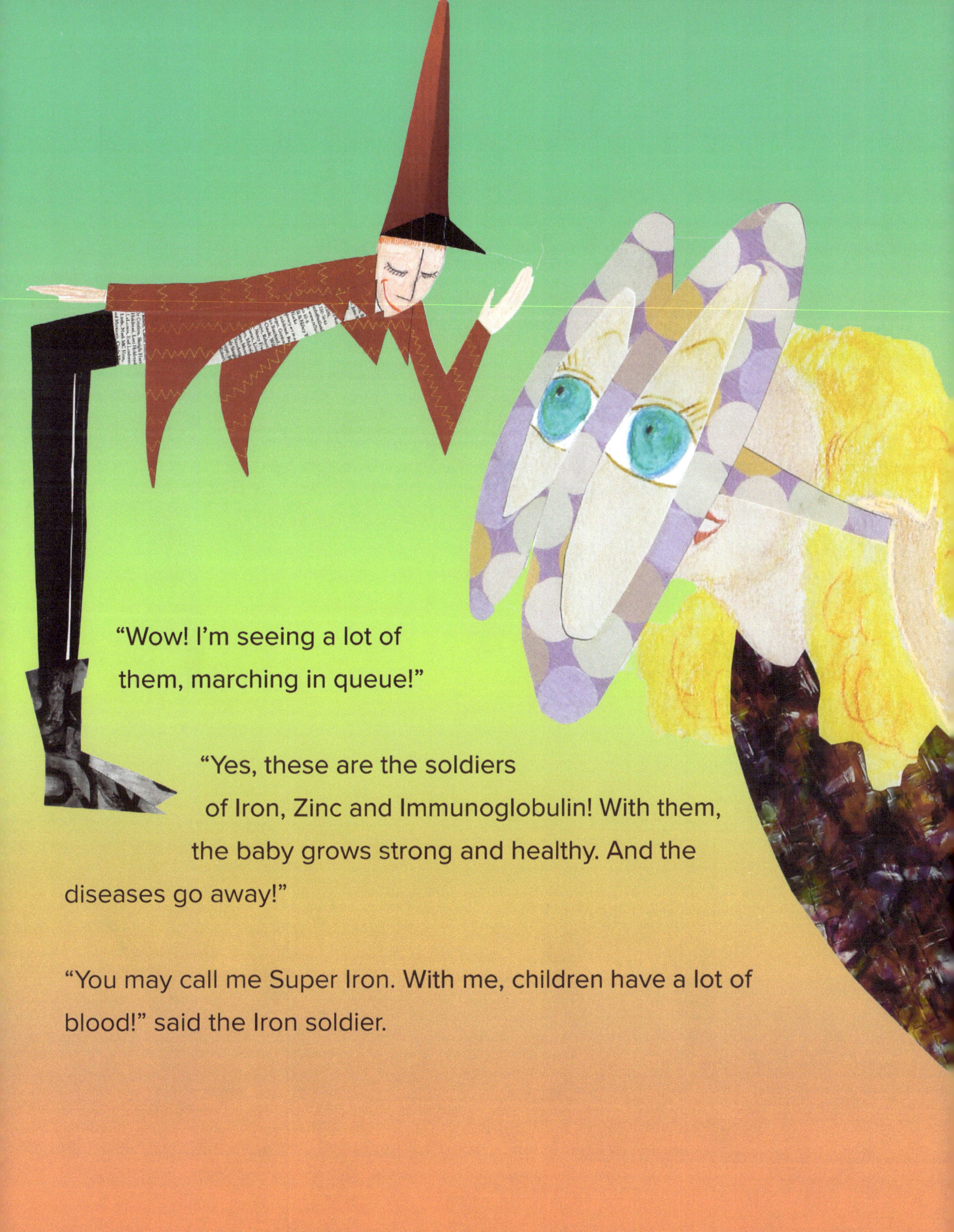

"Wow! I'm seeing a lot of them, marching in queue!"

"Yes, these are the soldiers of Iron, Zinc and Immunoglobulin! With them, the baby grows strong and healthy. And the diseases go away!"

"You may call me Super Iron. With me, children have a lot of blood!" said the Iron soldier.

"I am Zin, and this is Glob, we both defend the body against diseases!" said the Zinc soldier.

"Nice to meet you!" Ana replied.

"This is Cal, the Calcium soldier. He is a sleepyhead, and needs the sunlight to march with all of us!"

"Ahhh! And this is why they take Kaeu to the playground in the morning?"

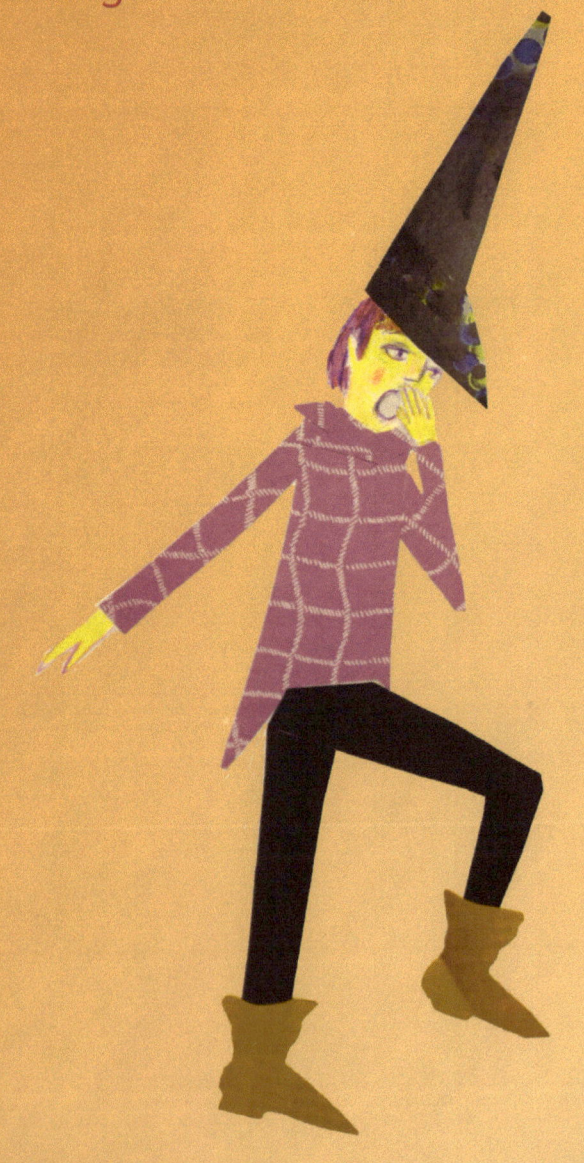
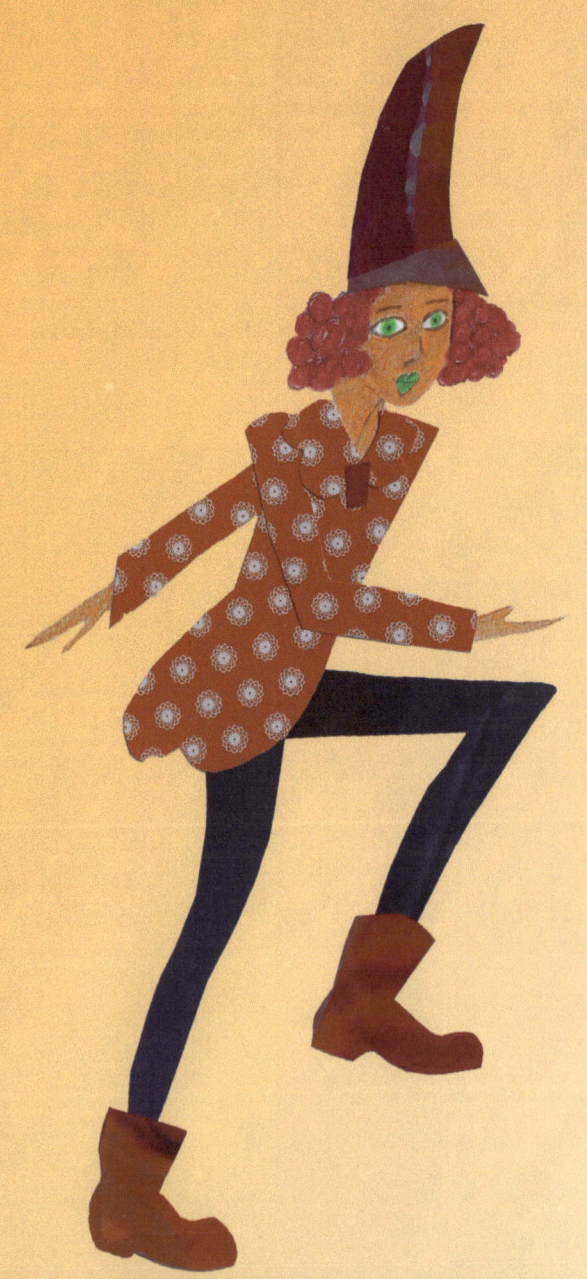

"Of course, you are so smart! The sun helps his body to absorb calcium, which is very important for our bones! This is true for everyone: from babies to old people."

Ana, increasingly interested, asked Aunt Deb:

"Does he only drink milk?"

"Sure, breast milk is the best food for babies up to 6 months."

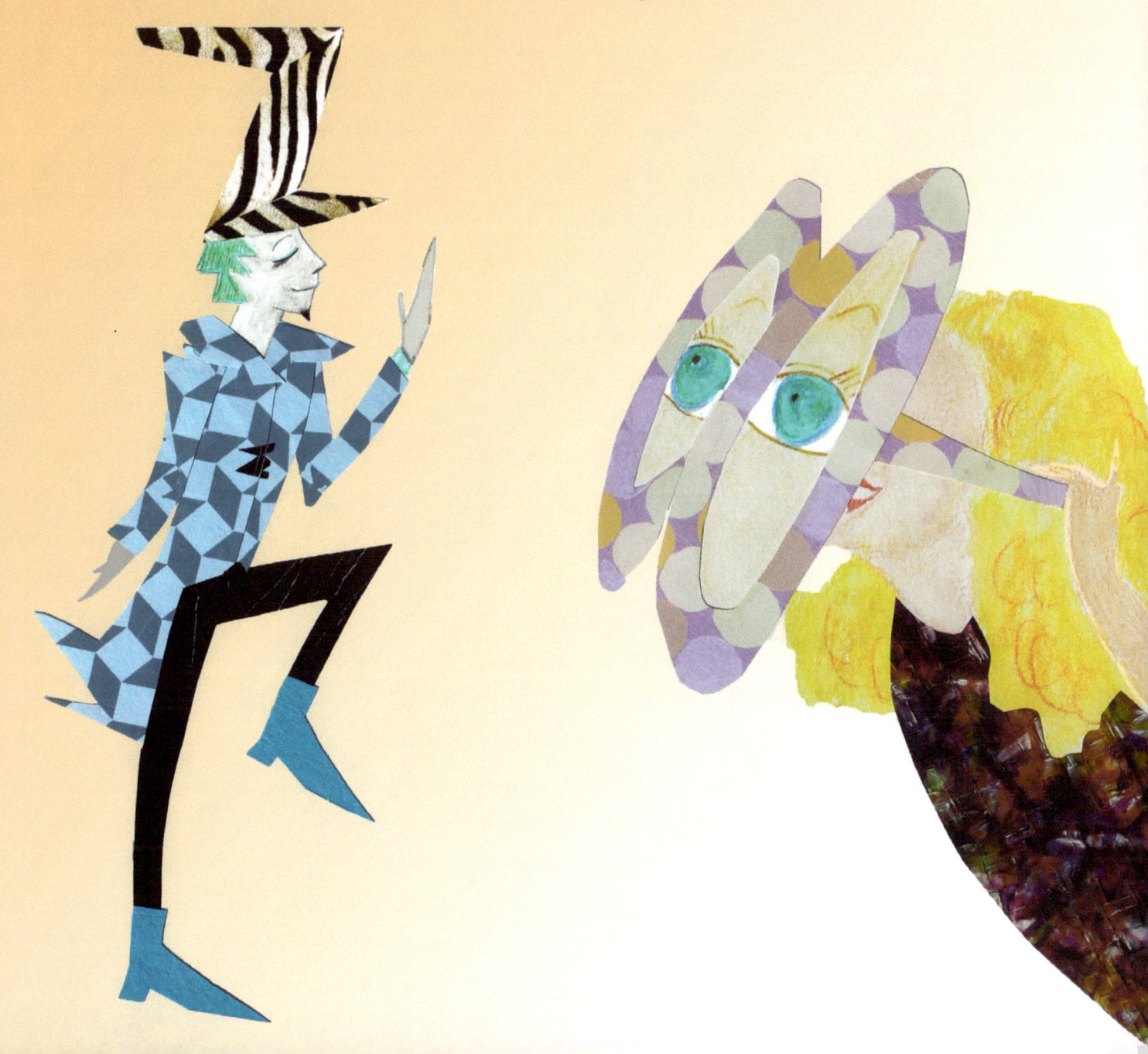

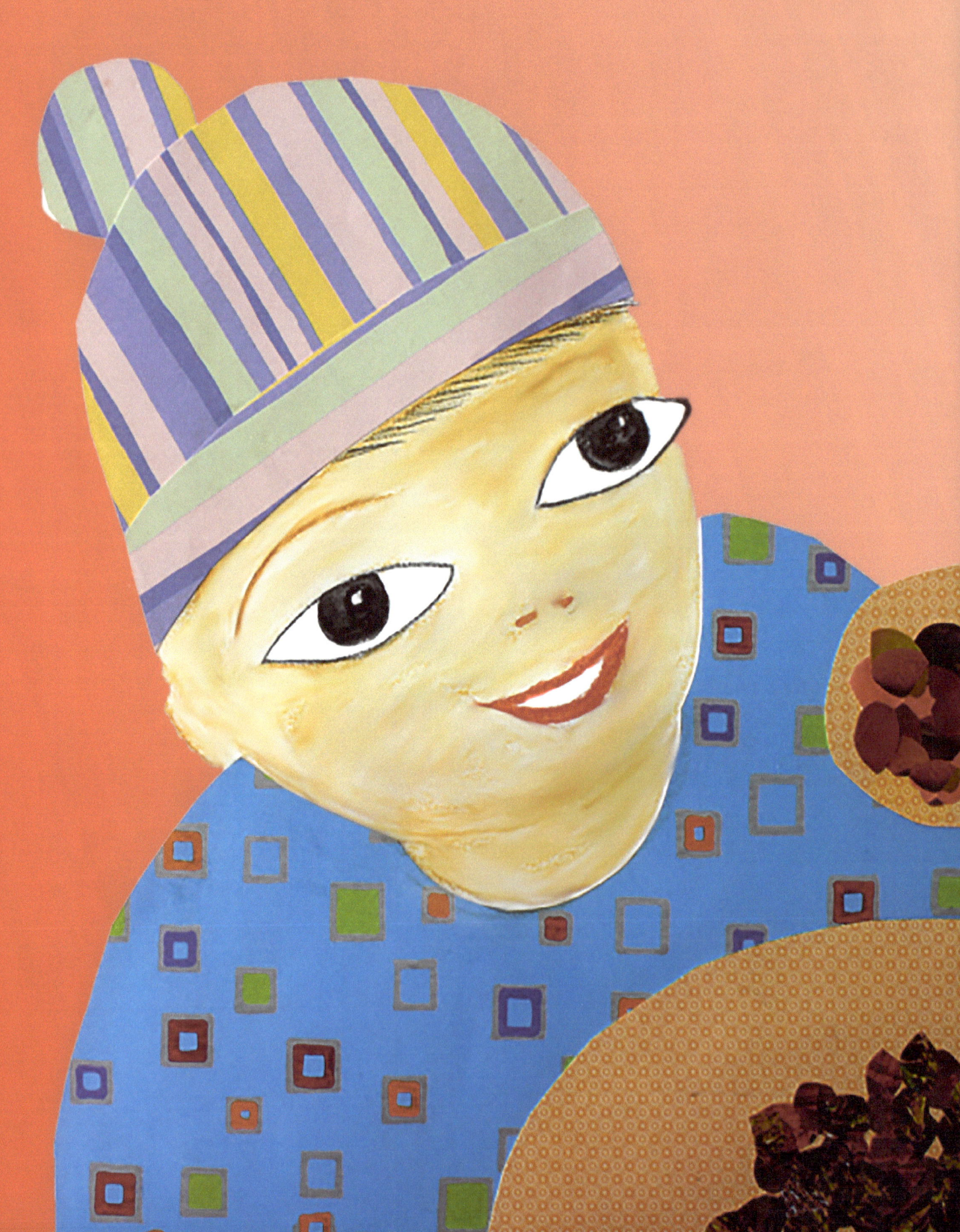

"And then?"

"As the baby grows, the number of soldiers decreases. And if he does not have the little soldiers, Sadie, the witch, comes back bringing diseases. For this reason, the mother should offer other types of food between feedings, as pureed meat and fortified cereal. Would you like to see how the colors bring joy to our body?"

"YES!!!"

"Let's cook!" Aunt Deb said.

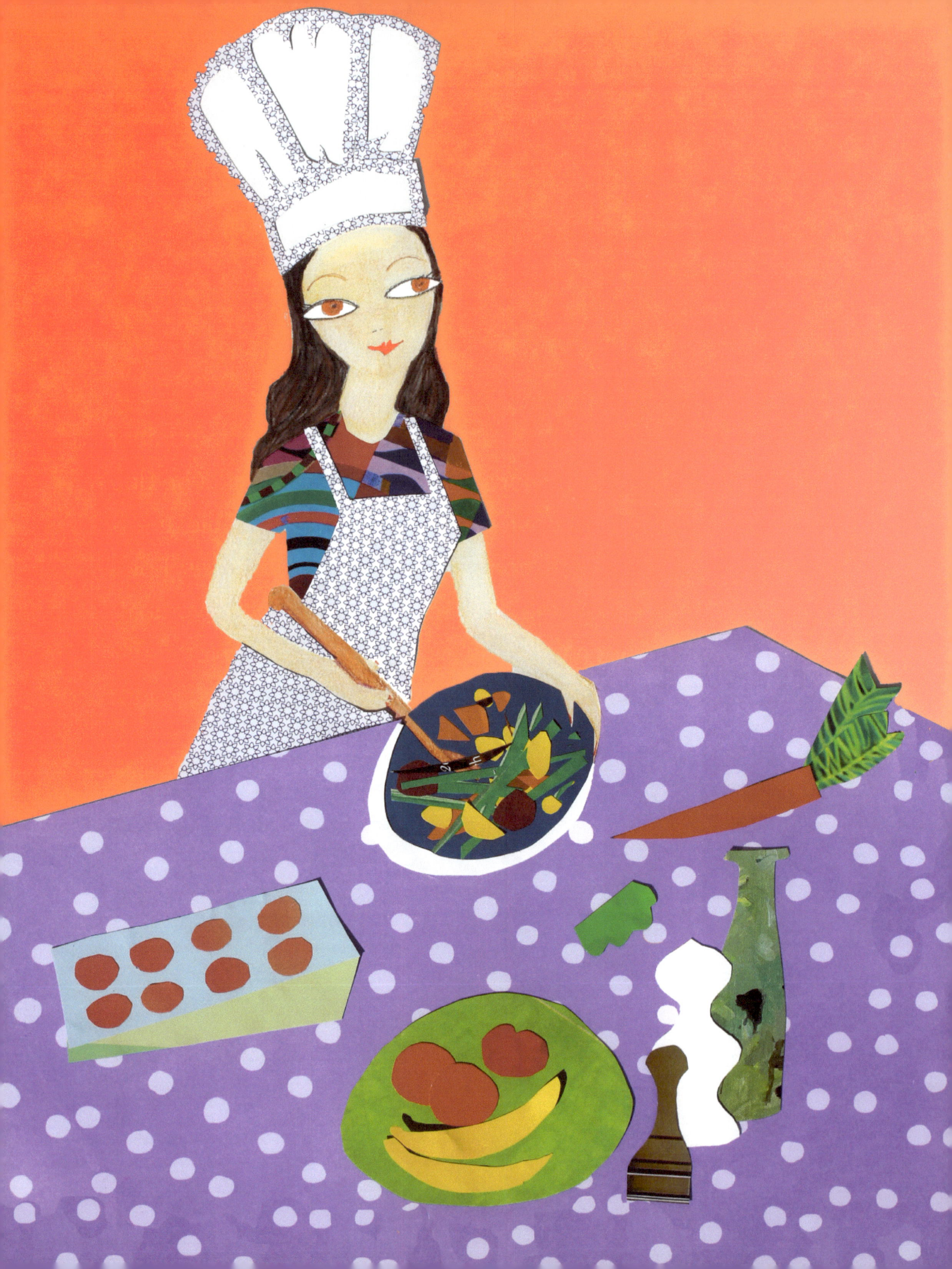

Ana and Aunt Deb went to the kitchen to prepare colorful and nutritious recipes.

Ana was impressed! Her Aunt could play so many roles in her life! As a charming Aunt Deb, or as a very smart and mighty doctor, and now there she was as a chef, ready for prepare the most beautiful meals in the world!

"Aunt Deb, I have a great idea! Let's invite other children to learn about all these colorful foods!"

"Awesome!" Aunt Deb cheered. "We are going to write down the recipes, so everyone will be able to discover the Fun World of colorful food".

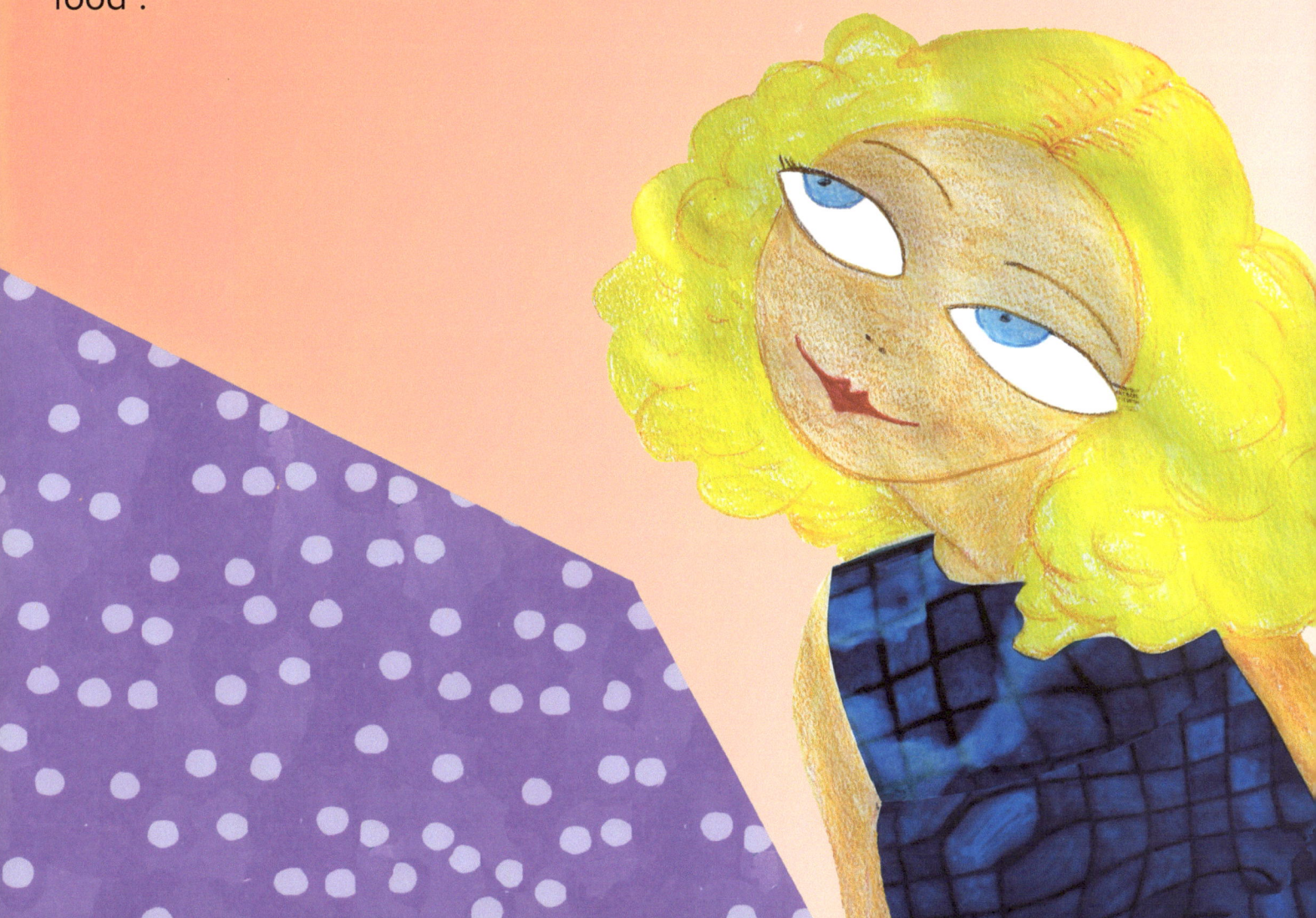

Zucchini Omelet

Ingredients for one serving:

1 beaten egg

1 cup of zucchini, grated (or broccoli, corn, carrots or any other vegetable)

3 cherry tomatoes

2 fresh basil leaves

Heat a nonstick skillet over medium heat. Stir-fry the grated zucchini (you may use corn, broccoli, carrots or any other vegetable). Add the beaten egg. Decorate the omelet using the tomatoes for the eyes and nose, and fresh basil leaves for the mouth.

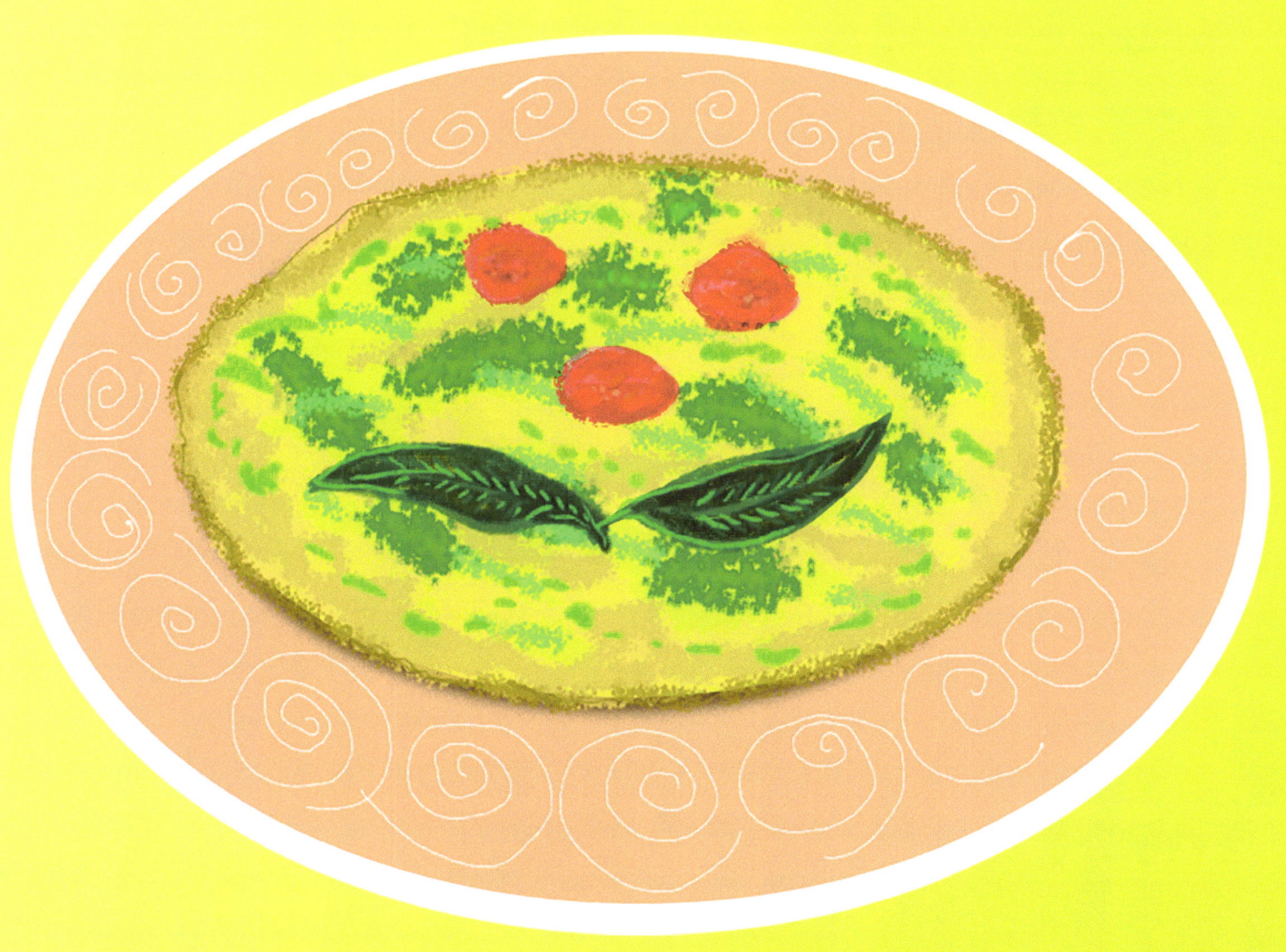

Quinoa Waffle

Ingredients for one serving:

1 ready-to- eat gluten free quinoa waffle

1 tomato slice

1 tablespoon of ricotta cheese

1 poached egg (Break the egg into a saucer, and then simmer it into boiling water for 2 minutes)

Spread the ricotta cheese on top of the quinoa waffle; add a tomato slice, and finally a poached egg. To make a sweet version, substitute yogurt for the ricotta cheese, substitute red fruits for the poached egg, and top it all with honey and a pinch of cinnamon.

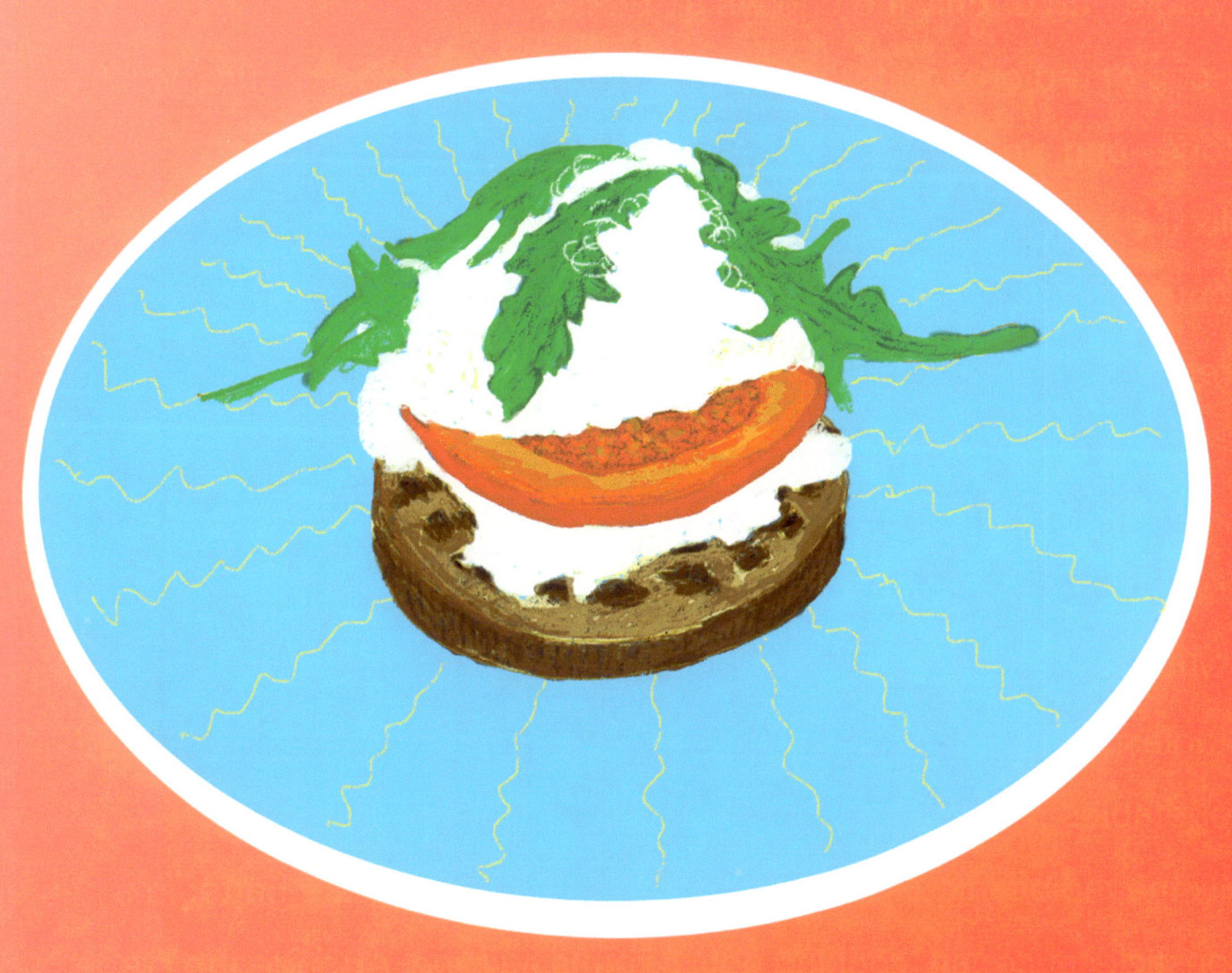

Tapioca Crepe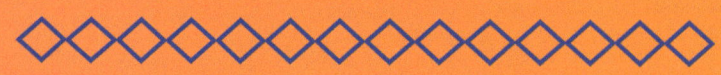

Sweet Version

Ingredients for one serving:

1 tablespoon of tapioca flour

1 whole egg or only the egg white, beaten

½ cup of red organic fruits (cherry, strawberry, raspberry, etc.), washed

Honey and cinnamon to taste

Mix the tapioca flour with the beaten egg and place the batter in a heated nonstick saucepan, cooking until it forms a crepe. Arrange the crepe in a plate, top it with the fruit, honey and cinnamon and fold it in half.

Salted Version

Ingredients for one serving:

1 tablespoon of tapioca flour

1 whole egg or only the egg white, beaten

1 tablespoon of cheese, cooked, shredded chicken or cooked, diced vegetables

Mix the tapioca flour with the beaten egg and place the batter in a heated nonstick saucepan, cooking until it forms a crepe. Arrange the crepe in a plate, top it with the cheese, shredded chicken or cooked vegetables and fold it in half.

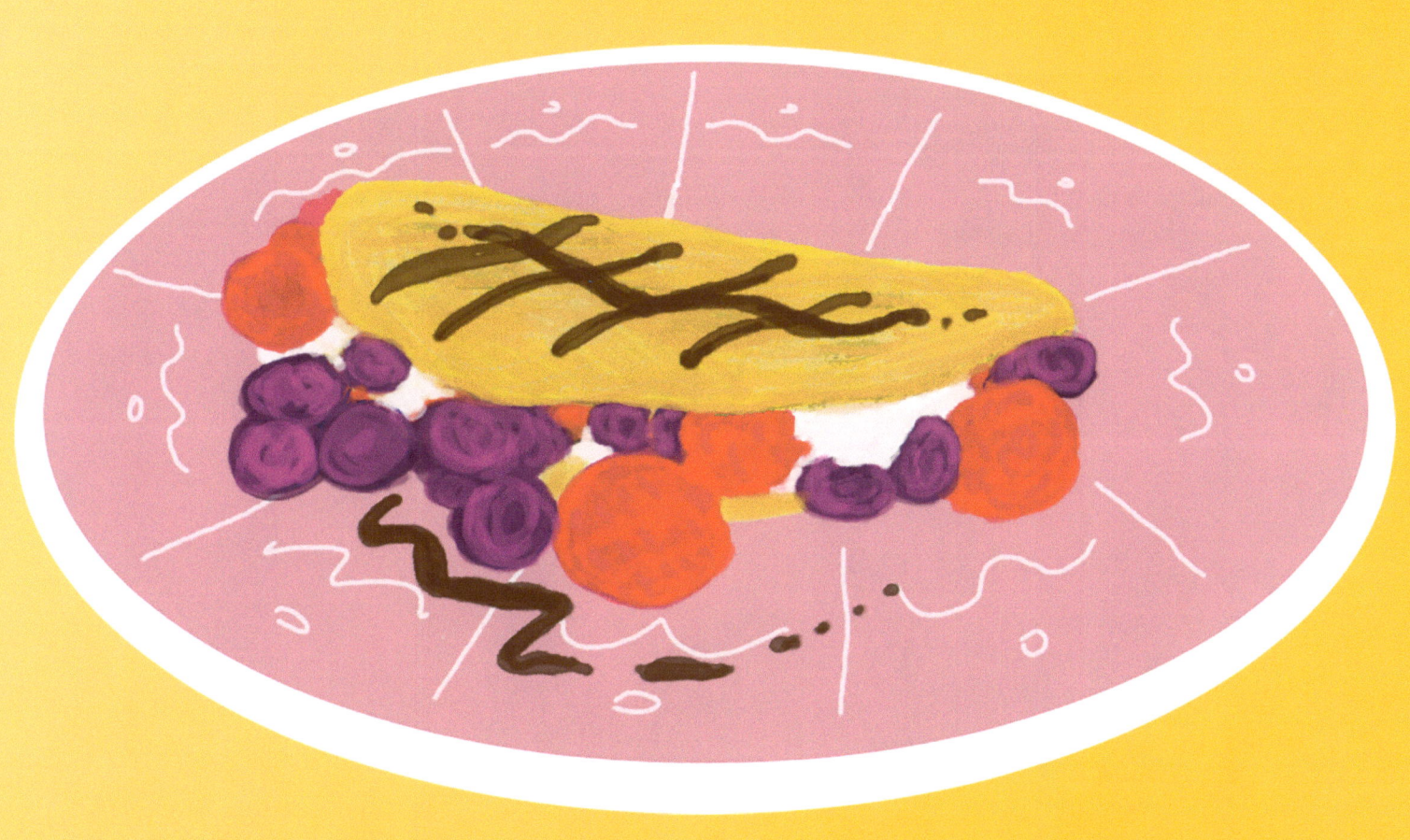

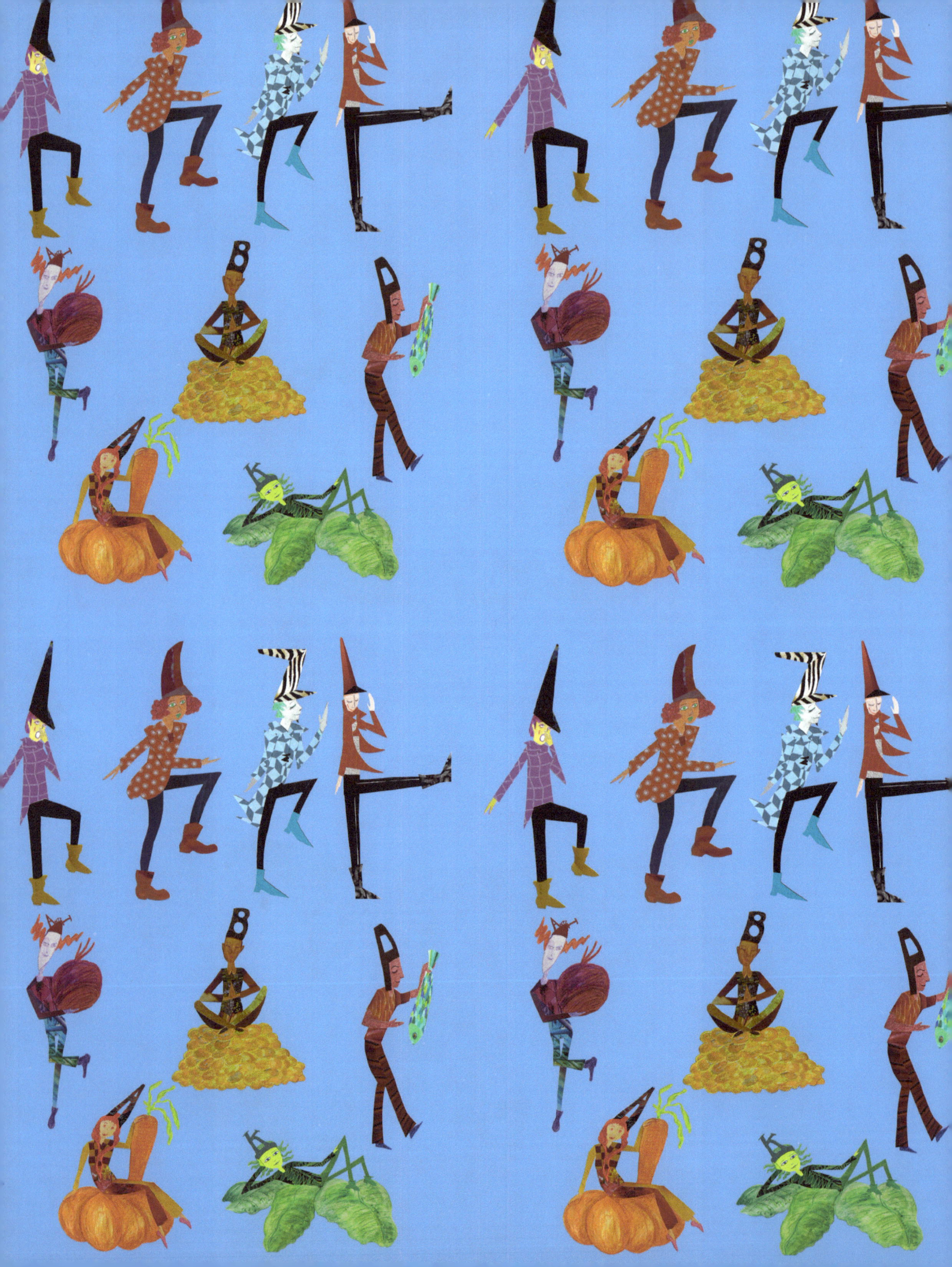